Healing Hepatitis C
with Modern Chinese Medicine

Qingcai Zhang, M.D.

Sino-Med Institute
420 Lexington Avenue, Graybar Building, Suite 631
New York, NY 10170

Published by Sino-Med Institute
420 Lexington Avenue, Graybar Building, Suite 631
New York, NY 10170, USA
Tel: 212-573-9584   Fax: 212-573-6639
Web site: http://www.sinomedresearch.org
Products information: http://hepahealth.com
Call 1-888-788-4372 toll-free.

First Printing: May 2000

Library of Congress Cataloging-in-Publication Data
ISBN 0-96772136-9

This publication is based on my personal research and clinical experience. The material is not intended to be used to diagnose or treat viral hepatitis. It is for informational and educational purposes only. If you think you may have hepatitis or have been diagnosed with hepatitis, consult your physician or healthcare practitioner.

Healing Hepatitis C with Modern Chinese Medicine
Includes index:
1. Hepatitis C (Disease). 2. Modern Chinese Medicine.
3. Case Studies. 4. Clinical Data.
I. Nye, Heidi. II. Title

Table of Contents

Acknowledgements i

Preface iii

Chapter 1: Healing Hepatitis C with Modern
             Chinese Medicine 1

Chapter 2: Chinese Herbal Therapeutics for
             Hepatitis C 31

Chapter 3: Clinical Therapeutics for Hepatitis C-
             Related Conditions 40

Chapter 4: Herbal Remedies and Their
             Pharmacology 45

Chapter 5: Frequently Asked Questions 87

Chapter 6: Case Studies — Patient Stories 101

Appendix   The Efficacy of Zhang's Chinese
             Herbal Protocol in Treating
             Hepatitis C: A Retrospective
             Analysis of its Clinical Practice 120

Glossary 130

Index 136

Acknowledgements

I could not have published this book without the help and encouragement of my friends, colleagues, patients, and family members. First, Andrew Weil, MD, whose recommendations focused my clinical and research work on hepatitis C, and Susan Piver, who read the manuscript and provided her views as both a patient and a friend. Many other patients commented on my theories and approaches, including John S, Linda S, Joseph V, and Vivian K. Matthew Dolen, author of *The Hepatitis C Handbook*, spoke with me regarding the main points of this book when he visited my New York office in the summer of 1998.

I presented review copies to the World Class Brainstorming Team's first conference of the Hepatitis C Caring Ambassadors Program, held in San Diego in December 1999. Review copies were also presented to Dr. Andrew Weil and two of his students, Drs. Monica Stokes and Opher Caspi of the Program in Integrative Medicine at the University of Arizona. They spent precious time reading and critiquing the manuscript. My friend and former English teacher Susan Gardos did an initial edit and her husband, Professor Howard Bleich, MD, of Harvard Medical School, read sections of the manuscript. My clinical colleague, Cyril Khanyile, MD, tested the herbal protocols on his patients and gave me valuable feedback as to how to make improvements. My friend and former employer Daniel Hsu, president of Brion Herbs Corporation, provided suggestions on enhancing the text. Tonya Bishoff's extensive corrections and suggestions have clarified this book. Heidi Nye, who also served as editor of my two previous books on AIDS and Chinese medicine, was the editor of this book. I thank her for improving the readability of the text and for her close attention to detail. Finally, my wife, Lily, and my son, Yale, were extremely supportive of the HepaPro Corporation of California, which makes my herbal products and this book available to hepatitis patients via the mail. In truth, my practice, my research, and my writing would hold little meaning without the love of my family.

Preface

When I began researching and treating HIV infection with modern Chinese medicine in 1987, I found that chronic viral diseases have been very difficult for pharmaceuticals to treat. True, smallpox and polio—two viral diseases—have been virtually eradicated, but with vaccines, not medications. Vaccination strengthens the immune system, enabling it to prevent and fight off viral infections. A healthy immune function is the most important factor in warding off viral infections.

HIV is the most medicated chronic viral infection in medical history, but to date not a single case has been cured. In the late '80s mono-therapy (such as AZT, d4t, and DDI) was used, though it proved unsuccessful because HIV quickly developed resistance. In the mid '90s, in order to avoid rapid resistance, combination treatments were developed using three or four drugs simultaneously. This breakthrough helped many patients lower their HIV load in the blood. Many patients became healthier, and their life span and quality of life improved. The price, however, was often high—severe side effects, including liver damage. Many patients exhibited enlarged stomachs, elevated levels of liver enzymes, jaundice, and fat deposits. Moreover, the HIV continues to mutate and resist this aggressive drug regimen. Today the conventional medical establishment is considering the use of so-called "kitchen sink therapy," whereby seven or eight drugs are used concurrently. One wonders how patients will be able to tolerate this regimen.

Last May, researchers from Johns Hopkins University reported that even with these strong medicines, the HIV hides in the memory cells of the immune system for about 60 years. This means that only relying on medications to fight off viral infections is not the answer.

In the development of protocols for hepatitis C treatment, the conventional medical establishment often follows in the footsteps of the HIV experience: first, using alpha interferon as mono-therapy, then adding ribavirin as a combination therapy. And protease inhibitors are under development. I believe this approach will not work well, since its major side effect is liver damage. It is not rational to use a treatment that damages the liver to treat the liver.

Why does the conventional medical establishment follow this approach? I think this is a paradigmatic problem. Conventional medicine was very successful in fighting bacterial infections with antibiotics. This success established its predominant position in the medical world. But viruses are very different from bacteria. Bacteria are independent living things and can reproduce without the host's participation. Using antibiotics to kill them does not greatly harm the host. Viruses, on the other hand, are dependent living things. They become a part of the host they infect. Their replication requires the host's participation. Using drugs to interfere with their replication will eventually harm the host. Thus, the bacterial-infection paradigm is not suitable for viral infections.

After millions of years of human evolution, our bodies have developed mechanisms to fight viruses. In the case of HCV infection, during the first six months (acute infection stage), about 15% of patients spontaneously eradicate the virus from their bodies. Obviously, it is the immune system that is responsible for this eradication. On August 19, 1999, the *New England Journal of Medicine* published a survey done by the Centers for Disease Control. This article reported that about 4.5 million Americans have been infected with HCV, 1.2 million (26%) of whom have cleared the HCV from their bodies. In other words, our body has the mechanism (the immunity) to eradicate the HCV. We should bolster the actions of our immune system to fight viral diseases and not try to take over or disturb this function. We should respect our body and its healing power.

Viral infection is a dynamic process. Both the virus and the infected body experience changes. Under the pressure of our immune system, the HCV can gradually mutate and become less harmful. At the same time, our immune system learns how to coexist with the virus and then how to control and eradicate it. I have seen some of our HIV patients reach the stage where they are totally healthy, although they may still have HIV in their bodies. Recently, two of my HIV patients reported to me that, when tested, the HIV was undetectable in their blood. They have never used any chemical drugs, only the herbs I prescribed for them. It takes five to ten years to reach this state. Another of my patients still tested HIV positive, but has never been sick, and his blood chemical panel has never been abnormal. He enjoys a completely normal and healthy life. These three patients were all diagnosed with HIV more than 15 years ago. This experience tells me that it is possible to coexist with the virus and keep it at bay. Mine is a realistic approach to fighting chronic viral infections. In this course of coexistence and control of the virus, the medicinal herbal remedies regulate immunity and suppress the potency of the virus.

My herbal protocol has effectively improved more than 80% of my viral hepatitis patients' conditions, enabling them to resume normal or near-normal life quality and life expectancy. Many patients and their conventional doctors have often asked me, if the herbs are so good, why are my remedies not tested by double-blind, placebo-controlled randomized tests and accepted by the medical world? To conduct such tests requires a prohibitive amount of money, manpower, and time. In private practice, it is impossible for me to conduct these tests. Furthermore, language and cultural barriers make it difficult for the conventional medical establishment to understand Chinese medicine and to conduct these trials.

My thoughts are daily stimulated by my conventional counterparts. Patients bring me all kinds of reactions from their conventional doctors. I have to spend a lot of time explaining the differences between Chinese and Western medicine to my patients.

The difference between my approach and the conventional one is in our way of thinking. Conventional medicine reduces a complicated disease like hepatitis C to a virus, then focuses its therapy solely on eradicating the virus. In contrast, I use traditional Chinese medicine (TCM) principles that see viral hepatitis as a complicated disease in which the virus is merely the factor that initiates the condition. After the disease develops during its long chronic course, many constitutional changes—immune dysfunction, liver damage, bile retention, fibrosis, and portal vein hypertension—can affect the disease course. Sometimes these factors have deeper and more profound effects on the disease development than the virus itself does. Treating viral hepatitis by only dealing with the virus is woefully insufficient.

Another difference between Chinese and Western medicine is that the former focuses on health rather than disease. It focuses on keeping the body in balance and believes that a well-balanced body can fight pathogens much more effectively than a body that is already impaired. In TCM, this principle is called "support the right and dispel evil." So, in treating chronic viral hepatitis, the most important task is to restore normal liver function and the overall health of the patient. With the aid of herbal remedies, a healthier body can coexist with the HCV and eventually eradicate it.

Hepatitis C is a relatively new disease. It was only defined a little more than 10 years ago. Many aspects of this disease are still unknown and require further research. My approach to its treatment is unlike the conventional approach, and many of my opinions will not mesh with my conventional counterparts. I consider this an asset, since looking at something from a different angle often provides new insights and even breakthroughs. This book encompasses my research to date, but it will not end here. It is ongoing, always seeking to develop better treatments for hepatitis C.

1

Healing Hepatitis C with Modern Chinese Medicine

What can you expect from this book?

When you open this book, I assume that you are looking for something unconventional. Please be prepared to read alternative views about treating hepatitis C. Different views can lead to different approaches, thereby producing different results. My view is derived from my practice of treating viral diseases with modern Chinese medicine. I have treated people with chronic viral infections, such as HIV, herpes, and hepatitis C for more than 13 years. I will introduce you to a foreign medical system with a different philosophy of dealing with hepatitis C — and explain how and why this medical system can be a complement of conventional Western medicine.

For whom is this book written?

First, this book is for those already diagnosed with hepatitis C. It will provide these patients with a different perspective on

their condition. Second, it is for the loved ones of these
patients, since it endeavors to instill them with the confidence
that their loved ones can be healed from this liver disease.
Third, it is for conventional medical practitioners who may
have referred patients to me. I hope to share my knowledge
and experience with them regarding my treatment of their
patients and the methodology behind it. Fourth, for the
general public, I would like to offer hepatitis C as an example
of what modern Chinese medicine is and how it can be used in
conjunction with conventional Western medicine. Integrating
Western and Chinese medicine is one way of creating more
effective treatments.

Why am I publishing this book?

Much coverage of hepatitis C has appeared lately in the
news media. Almost every major television network, magazine,
and newspaper has covered this disease. Most of these stories
are terrifying and inflammatory, calling hepatitis C the "shadow
epidemic" and "the next AIDS," emphasizing its bleakest prognosis.

An article appearing in the *New Yorker* (May 11, 1998),
"The Shadow Epidemic," was written by an authoritative doctor, the chairman of a committee making recommendations to
the Food and Drug Administration (FDA) for alpha interferon, proposed as a treatment for hepatitis C. The conclusion
of the article is extremely pessimistic: "We (the patient and the
doctor) sat for a while in silence and agreed that there was
only one choice: to wait and hope that medical science will
move more quickly than the course of her infection." The committee knew that "there was no evidence that interferon treatment would save lives, but we were aware of the lack of any

alternative (emphasis added), and of the desperate needs of hepatitis C patients for relief. The drug could provide a respite from the virus for several months, and might, so we hoped, also slow the march to cirrhosis and death. Seven years later, the options for treatment have barely changed."

I was hurt by this attitude—not only because I am a Chinese medical practitioner, but also because I feel that such an attitude prevents many hepatitis C sufferers from obtaining effective treatments from other medical systems. Patients don't want to read articles that make them fearful and lose their will to fight the disease. The more they read, the more depressed they become. This is the very reason I am writing this book— to proclaim that there are effective alternative medicines available to viral hepatitis patients.

Many of my patients encouraged me to write this book so that more people will know that they don't have to wait and suffer. Means exist to help them get healthier.

What is the significance of hepatitis C?

Viral hepatitis, especially hepatitis C, is currently the most prevalent infectious disease in the U.S. More than 4.5 million Americans have been infected with hepatitis C, and 2.7 million currently carry the hepatitis C virus. More than 30,000 new cases are diagnosed each year. Hepatitis C is an insidious, stealthy virus that mutates while hiding within liver and other organ cells, making it very difficult for the body's immune system to eradicate it. Additionally, hepatitis C tends to progress slowly over many years (20 to 30), resulting in as many as 74% of infected patients having few noticeable symptoms until they reach an advanced chronic stage. Hepatitis C results in 8,000 to 10,000 deaths annually. It is also the leading cause for liver transplants in the U.S. Without effective treatment, this figure is expected to triple within the next 10 to 20 years.

As the disease progresses, blood tests indicate elevated liver enzyme levels (ALT, AST), which are indicative of liver damage and inflammation. As the course of the disease gradually disrupts crucial liver functions, it progresses to cirrhosis (scarring), which, in a small portion of patients, can then lead to hepatocellular carcinoma, a type of primary liver cancer.

Although the severity of hepatitis C is much less than HIV infection, four times as many people are infected with HCV than HIV. Hepatitis C causes more morbidity (sickness) than mortality (death). It has a much slower disease course, therefore, we have more time to treat and alter its course. Since it affects the lives of so many people, there is a great need to develop effective treatments that can fight this disease. Chinese medicine is an effective way to do so.

What is traditional Chinese medicine?

Traditional Chinese medicine (TCM) is an important part of Chinese culture. China is one of the oldest civilizations in the world. Its long history has produced a unique culture, which, in turn, has produced a unique medicine—TCM.

In the U.S., TCM is considered an alternative medicine, but in China it is mainstream. This complete, well-documented medical system can be briefly described in three words: ancient, comprehensive, and new.

1. TCM is ancient.

TCM is a very old, but vital health and healing system based on harmony or balance. A healthy person is in complete harmony, both internally and with nature. China's first physicians were also philosophers, and their medical theories were deeply rooted in Taoism. *Huang Di Nei Jin* (The Yellow Emperor's Classic of Internal Medicine), compiled more than 2,000 years ago, laid down the principles of TCM. The Chinese medical sage Zhang Zhongjing formulated TCM's clinical therapeutics about 1,800 years ago. He set them forth in *Shang Han Lun* (Treatise on Febrile Diseases) and *Jin Gau Yao Lue* (Prescriptions from the Golden Chamber) —still used today by TCM practitioners.

Like most traditional medicine, TCM developed mainly through clinical observation, so it is empirically based. It uses inductive methods to summarize clinical experience and instruct further practice. TCM developed such unique diagnostic and therapeutic methods as tongue diagnosis, pulse reading, herbal formulas, acupuncture, tui-na (Chinese style massage), and qi-gong (breathing exercise) to treat patients holistically. Over the centuries, TCM has continued to evolve, most recently with scientifically conducted clinical trials and pharmacological studies of herbal preparations.

2. TCM is comprehensive.

TCM is a comprehensive medical system that serves more than a billion people in Asia, with more than a million TCM practitioners in China alone. In Japan, more than 200,000 physicians prescribe Chinese herbal medicine for their patients. Five years ago, the Chinese government conducted a nationwide survey on Chinese materia medica and found that more than 12,000 plants, animal products, and minerals have been used as TCM remedies. TCM treats almost every disease identified by modern Western medicine, and recently TCM has spread to many Western countries. It was developed in China, an area as big as Europe, and is used today by nearly one-quarter of the world's population. We can safely say that TCM is the second largest medical system in the world.

3. TCM is new.

TCM also offers a modern approach to healthcare. During the past four decades, a new phenomenon has occurred within TCM: the integration of TCM with modern Western medicine. This is a reflection of a feature of the Chinese culture: its great capacity to endure, contain, and assimilate foreign cultures. One such example is the introduction of Buddhism from India, its widespread acceptance by the Chinese people, and its eventual transformation into a Chinese version.

Modern Western medicine came to China about 150 years ago, and today is generally accepted by the Chinese people. Now a new phase of adaptation has begun—that of combining with indigenous Chinese medicine, thereby creating a new hybrid of integrated medicine. This happy marriage of TCM and modern Western medicine has brought great benefits to the patients it serves.

What is modern Chinese medicine?

The modernization movement brought TCM into every medical school in China, to be taught along with Western medicine. It has been practiced side by side with Western medicine by the same doctors for the same patients in the same medical settings. For most clinical conditions, these two medical approaches are used together, and the results are usually better than either would have achieved if used alone. As part of this movement, many Western-trained doctors have devoted tremendous amounts of time and energy to scientific studies of TCM, resulting in a new medicine—Integrative Chinese and Western Medicine (ICWM).

This movement has resulted in three kinds of medical practice in China: TCM, Western medicine, and ICWM. I prefer to call ICWM modern Chinese medicine (MCM).

How was Chinese medicine modernized?

One method used to modernize TCM was the creation of a terminology of pathophysiological diagnosis to match TCM's constitutional diagnosis and phytopharmacology (pharmacology of botanical products) to match the terms of Chinese herbology. In this way, language barriers between these two medical systems have gradually been overcome. Moreover, studies have shown TCM to be effective in treating newly discovered and newly defined diseases, such as HIV, Lyme disease, and hepatitis C. Although these diseases are not discussed in the classic texts of TCM, their pathophysiological and pharmacological descriptions can be used to research suitable TCM diagnoses and treatments.

Because of the development of phytopharmacology of Chinese materia medica, we now can use herbs based, not only on TCM principles, but on the active ingredients of the herbs, their physiological actions, the pharmakenics (metabolism) of their active ingredients in the body, their possible toxicity and adverse reactions, and appropriate clinical dosages and treatment courses. All these studies make MCM a more effective medicine than TCM. It can treat some newly defined diseases. Treating chronic viral hepatitis with MCM is a good example of this development.

How did I begin treating hepatitis C?

Since 1987, I have treated more than a thousand AIDS patients with Chinese medicine. AIDS patients have many complications and co-infections, and hepatitis C is a common co-infection. While treating HIV infection, I also treated many hepatitis C cases. HIV combination therapies resulted in drug-induced liver damage—highly elevated ALT, jaundice, and fat deposits in the liver and stomach. Both drug-induced liver damage and hepatitis C responded favorably to Chinese herbal treatment. Because of the encouraging clinical results our patients obtained, I began seeing more and more hepatitis C patients.

In 1995, John S was referred to me by his family physician, who treats some of the same hepatitis C patients I do. John contracted hepatitis C in 1983. Since his ALT was always high and his three liver biopsies showed mild fibrosis and chronic active inflammation, he was always very tired. After treatment with interferon failed, he began searching for alternative treatments. Two months after starting our herbal treatments, his liver enzyme levels normalized for the first time in 12 years, and his fatigue and pain in the liver area were gone. He underwent gallstone surgery in 1997. The surgeon found his liver to be much better than those of other patients with hepatitis C. Compared with previous biopsies, the new biopsy found the inflammation and fibrosis significantly reduced. John was so happy that he started writing letters to influential people in an attempt to spread the word that there is an alternative way to treat hepatitis C. One of the people he contacted was Dr. Andrew Weil, a renowned authority on alternative medicine. As fate would have it, John was on a train to Washington,

D.C., and happened to sit next to Dr. Weil. Since then, Dr. Weil has been referring patients to me, especially those with hepatitis C.

One of the patients Dr. Weil referred was his friend Susan Piver. She had contracted hepatitis C in 1985, when she received blood transfusions after a car accident. After consulting with two gastroenterologists, she was reluctant to take interferon, a drug with many side effects and a response rate of only around 20%. Dr. Weil suggested she see me for Chinese herbal treatment. When I first saw Susan, she was pale and weak, with a somber, white complexion with a blue-green tinge, and yellowish eyes. She was in constant pain in her liver area and often nauseated. She dragged through the workday. After three months on the Chinese herbs I prescribed for her, she had her liver-enzyme levels tested, and they were normal for the first time in 12 years. Six months later, in January 1998, her re-test remained normal. That was an extremely encouraging sign, and the results of the herbal treatment have been sustained. Her complexion became normal, her liver area pain disappeared, and her energy level improved. After about one year of herbal treatment, she told Dr. Weil, "I don't think of myself as someone with hepatitis anymore." Recently, she was married. My wife and I were invited to her wedding. Seeing Susan happy and healthy was one of the greatest rewards of my clinical work.

Dr. Weil related Susan's story in his article "Natural Help for Hepatitis," which was published in the April 1998 issue of his *Self Healing* newsletter. He put my name and address in that article. From this I received an overwhelming reader response. The first day this article was published, I received 574 letters. In about two months' time, I received more than

2,000 letters from people concerned about chronic hepatitis C and B. This showed that the need for alternative treatments for hepatitis C was indeed extremely urgent. Since then, I have treated more than 600 hepatitis C patients—the majority of whom have responded very well. Currently my practice is focused on hepatitis C, and I am doing extensive research to develop more effective herbal treatments for the disease.

How do conventional doctors react to my approach?

Doctors of conventional Western medicine respond differently to Chinese medicine. In the case of hepatitis C, doctors are often frustrated by the lack of effective treatments to offer their patients. A few of them, like Dr. Weil, who has great foresight and sagacity, have begun to advocate integrative medicine. Many doctors have listened to their patients' positive accounts of their experiences with Chinese medicine and have begun to look at this alternative. Some doctors want to know what I give our patients. Some even write letters to recommend my treatments. Some tell their patients, "If this is working for you, keep doing it."

There are also negative reactions and skepticism. The skepticism voiced against Chinese medicine did not surprise me. I myself had the same reaction when I was first introduced to TCM. I was in my third year of medical school and had already learned anatomy, histology, biochemistry, and pathology. Suddenly, the school started to teach us yin and yang, the Five Elements Theory, and other TCM concepts. My classmates and I shared the same attitude—we rejected TCM outright. We didn't want to learn this "unscientific" medicine. Only when we went on to do clinical work did we find that it really

worked. Reflecting back on my own early skepticism and ultimate embracing of TCM, I can well understand the suspicion
of TCM by some Western-trained physicians.

I am a clinician and I respect good clinical outcomes.
Medical science is an application science, and the final judg-
ment is the clinical outcome. Doctors should respect the clinical results and not reject the medicine because it is based on a
different theoretical system. Especially for hepatitis C, the
treatment results are measured by lab tests, not just the
patients' feelings. "Feeling better" may be considered a
placebo effect, but lab tests are undeniably objective, hard
data.

What are the conventional treatments available for hepatitis C?

Presently, the FDA-approved conventional treatment is
alpha interferon (IFN). The response rate is low and long-
term remission is uncommon. Approximately 35 to 40% of
patients treated with IFN for a six-month period show normalization of liver enzyme levels, as well as a reduction of viral
load and of inflammation diagnosed by liver biopsy. Unfor-
tunately, this improvement is short-lived, as 60% suffer relapse
within months after IFN treatment is discontinued. Thus, only
15 to 20% of patients treated with IFN can expect remission
for an unspecified time. Additionally, the side effects of IFN
can be quite severe—persistent "flu-like" symptoms, fatigue,
muscle aches, depression, headache, dizziness, general malaise,
insomnia, poor appetite, bone marrow depletion, hair loss, ir-
ritability, and even auto-immune diseases. The side effects of
IFN can be worse than the disease.

A new combination therapy, Rebetron, has recently been approved by the FDA. It is a combination of IFN and ribavirin, a nucleoside analogue (in the same family as AZT) developed in the late 1980s. It showed poor results when used alone for hepatitis C, though when combined with IFN in clinical trials, the combination therapy showed about a 50% sustained HCV suppression after the therapy stopped. However, it is much too soon to say that this is a good combination. Nucleoside analogue is a chemotherapy that is hard on the liver. The side effects of Rebetron can be dangerous. In addition to the IFN side effects mentioned above, ribavirin may produce birth defects and severe anemia that can lead to heart attack or stroke in those with risk factors. Psychiatric problems, such as suicidal tendencies, have also been reported.

What are the shortcomings of conventional treatments?

1. Conventional treatments might not be consistent with the first principle of medicine: DO NO HARM. Some of its side effects may be even more harmful than the disease itself.

2. Most patients I see have suffered with the disease for 20 to 30 years. At this stage, pathogenetic factors can have more profound effects on disease progression than the etiologic factor (the HCV). But conventional treatment is focused solely on the etiologic factor and does not address complicated chronic liver disease.

3. Conventional treatment interferes with immune function and can even cause auto-immune diseases, thereby further compromising the patient's health, since a healthy immune system is required for fighting the HCV.

4. Conventional treatments can only bring down the HCV load in about 50% of treated patients to an "undetectable" level in the blood. "Undetectable" is not synonymous with "total eradication", and upon checking the liver for these responders, most patients will still have HCV in their liver. Relapse will happen at a later time.

5. With conventional treatment, many patients become sicker, not healthier.

Because the patients I see are mostly non-responders to conventional treatments, my criticism may be biased. I welcome criticism of my approach from my conventional counterparts. Criticism and counter-criticism can help improve both our protocols.

Hepatitis C questions that conventional medicine has not addressed

1. What about the 50+% non-responders?

Since the efficacy of the IFN treatments is only about 15 to 25%, and the response to combination treatments is about 40 to 50%, many patients treated with conventional medicine will not have a positive response.

2. What can be done for those contraindicated for IFN and Rebetron treatments?

The contraindicated conditions include: de-compensated cirrhosis, persistently normal ALT, active alcohol or illicit drug use, history of severe depression, cytopenias (low white blood cell count), hyperthyroidism, renal transplant, and convincing evidence of auto-immune disease. It should be noted that most patients with these conditions are in great need of treatment.

3. How do you help those who can't tolerate conventional treatment?

Because of the side effects of IFN and Rebetron treatments, about 10 to 40% of patients have to reduce their dosage, and 5 to 15% have to stop treatment completely. These people will not be aided by conventional medications for hepatitis C.

4. What happens after the response period?

For those who do respond to IFN and Rebetron, how long the response lasts is another question that needs to be answered. Side effects and high cost prevent the usage of IFN and Rebetron as long-term maintenance treatments.

5. What can be done about the pathological damage that has already been done by chronic hepatitis C?

The clinical symptoms are signs of liver damage. Conventional treatments do not address this problem. So, people will naturally ask:

6. Is there an alternative way to treat hepatitis C?

Ancient civilizations developed their own medical systems, and they have dealt with hepatitis throughout their long histories. TCM has an abundance of literature on liver diseases.

Is there an alternative way to treat hepatitis C?

Due to the limited treatment protocol within conventional medicine, many patients are searching for alternatives. In the *New Yorker* magazine (May 11, 1998), Dr. Jerome Groopman wrote in "The Shadow Epidemic": "We were aware of the lack of any alternative..." "...there was only one choice: to wait..."

To this article, Dr. Andrew Weil responded: "Jerome Groopman, in 'The Shadow Epidemic,' makes no mention of the fact
that treatments other than interferon and ribavirin are available to patients with hepatitis C. In particular, modern
Chinese medical protocols using combinations of antiviral,
liver-protective, and anti-inflammatory herbs (all relatively
nontoxic) appear to halt the progression of the disease in
many cases. It would be easy to research the efficacy of such
therapy and compare it with the conventional regimen if ex-
perts were aware that the alternatives exist, and were open-
minded about integrating them into their practices." (May 18
1998, *New Yorker*)

In his newsletter, Dr. Weil went on to suggest that hepatitis
patients "try Chinese medicine":

"Doctors in China have a great deal of experience treating
hepatitis with traditional medicine (one-third of the world's
hepatitis carriers are in China), and Chinese studies show that
their herbal regime has a much higher sustained response rate
than the Western drug interferon, is more affordable, and has
no serious side effects..." ("Natural Help for Hepatitis," April
1998, *Self Healing*)

Why use Chinese medicine to treat hepatitis C?

A third of all hepatitis cases worldwide (of which 30 million
are hepatitis C) are found in China, with viral hepatitis being
the most prevalent infectious disease—10.3% of the Chinese
population are HBsAg positive, and more than 100 million are
HBsAg carriers. Every year, 10 million new cases are diagnosed. Chinese doctors treat most of the world's hepatitis
patients.

Because China is a developing country, expensive drugs, such as IFN and ribavirin, are not readily available, nor are they affordable. Therefore, Chinese doctors are mainly dependent on Chinese medicine to treat viral hepatitis. Chinese doctors employ an integrated approach in the treatment of hepatitis C and B. They use Western medicine's diagnostics together with Chinese medicine's constitutional differentiation and herbal treatments. Chinese herbal treatments suppress the HCV and HBV, regulate immunity, normalize liver enzyme levels, heal inflammation of liver cells, clear jaundice, improve the microcirculation of the liver, prevent fibrosis, and partially reverse cirrhosis.

A survey was done in China to compare Western and Chinese medicine for treating chronic viral hepatitis. It questioned 188 doctors from large city teaching hospitals and medium-sized city hospitals, as well as rural primary-care practitioners. Among them, 88 were Western medicine practitioners, 80 were TCM practitioners, and 20 were practitioners of integrative Chinese and Western medicine. All 188 doctors agreed that TCM and ICWM produce better therapeutic results in treating chronic viral hepatitis than does Western medicine.

How does Chinese medicine approach chronic viral infections?

Chinese medicine's approach is termed "*fu zheng qu xie*," literally translated as "dispel evil (the infectious agent) by supporting righteous qi (normal function of the body)." Following this principle, Chinese medicine has developed therapies to regulate the immune system. Chinese medicine is a constitutional medicine and purports that the body itself is the major healing force. Drugs and procedures can help to heal, but they cannot replace the healing function of the body. In the case of viral hepatitis, Chinese medicine first focuses on the normalization of liver function and the restoration of overall health. With improving health, the body's immune function is strengthened. Further, with the help of anti-viral herbal remedies, the HCV is suppressed and kept at bay, causing no further harm.

What are the clinical implications of the natural history of hepatitis C?

The statistical data on the natural history of hepatitis C is based on the National Institutes of Health's *Consensus Statement on Managing Hepatitis C*. From the data, we can see that hepatitis C progresses very slowly, which gives us time to treat and alter its disease course. In the acute stage (first six months), about 15% of patients will be able to resolve the infection spontaneously and recover completely. This means that the body has the mechanism (the immunity) to fight off HCV. The remaining 85% of infected persons will develop a chronic infection, though the majority of them (75%) will be stable. If the liver inflammation is well under control, this stability will last a very long time. About 25% of chronically infected patients will develop cirrhosis, but the majority of them (75%) will be stable. We can treat these people to partially reverse their fibrosis and keep them stable. Only 25% of those who have cirrhosis will progress to liver failure or liver cancer that will require a liver transplant. Overall, this population is only

5% of the total patients. This means that hepatitis C is much less serious than HIV and causes more morbidity (sickness) than mortality (death).

On August 19, 1999, the *New England Journal of Medicine* published the article "The Prevalence of Hepatitis C Virus Infection in the United States, 1988 Through 1994." This survey was done by the Centers for Disease Control and Prevention in Atlanta and found that "The overall prevalence of anti-HCV was 1.8%, corresponding to an estimated 3.9 million persons nationwide (95% confidence interval, 3.1 million to 4.8 million) with HCV infection....Seventy-four percent were positive for HCV RNA, indicating that an estimated 2.7 million persons in the United States (95% confidence interval, 2.4 million to 3.0 million) were chronically infected...." According to this report, at least 2.7 million Americans carry HCV, making it the most common infectious disease in the U.S.A. This is a conservative estimate; the actual number may be higher.

The most interesting thing to emerge from this report is that about 1.2 million people who were once infected no longer have any signs of the virus. These people eradicated the virus through their own disease-fighting power, i.e., their immunity. This further confirms that our body has the ability to eliminate the HCV. Previous data found only 15% of the patients can spontaneously eradicate the virus; now this proportion has increased to 26%. This is an encouraging figure. If we can help the other 74% restore their immune function, they might be able to do the same.

What is the ideal strategy for treating chronic hepatitis C?

1. Eradicate the virus or suppress replication of the virus.

2. Control liver inflammation and halt disease progression.

3. Suppress fibrosis and promote re-absorption of fibrotic tissue.

4. Promote regeneration of liver cells and restore liver function.

5. Turn chronic active hepatitis into chronic persistent hepatitis, then effect a clinical and histological cure.

Right now, we are still not able to reach all these goals. A comprehensive approach is needed to treat chronic viral hepatitis, including proper herbal treatment, rest, and nutrition. By doing this, we can at least halt progression of the disease and restore general health.

How can one distinguish between chronic active and chronic persistent hepatitis?

Some physicians have stopped using these terms, even though distinguishing clinically between CAH and CPH has important diagnostic, therapeutic, and prognostic significance. CAH is the type of chronic hepatitis that is actively progressing and is on a faster track to cirrhosis than CPH. Treatments must attempt to turn CAH to CPH and then to halt the progression. The following chart gives a comparison.

	CAH	CPH
Disease Course	>6 months	>6 months
Symptoms		
fatigue, anorexia, stomach distention, loose stool	Multiple	Few
Physical Signs	Obvious	Mild
enlarged & hardened liver & spleen, jaundice, bleeding, grayish complexion, liver palm, spider mole, edema		
Extra-liver Signs	Often	Few
joint pain, skin rashes, fever, thyroid inflammation, vasculitis, ulcerative colitis, Sjögren's syndrome, nephritis glomerular		
Liver Function Tests		
ALT	>150	<150
Gamma-globulin	elevated	not elevated
Bilirubin total	>1.5	<1.5
Pt time	prolonged	not prolonged
Auto-immune	ANA, AMA (+)	(-)
Histology	necrosis, inflammatory-cell infiltration in portal areas, lobe invasion, connective tissue hypertrophy, fibroblastic activities	no necrosis, mild inflammation, no lobe changes, signs of healing, no worse on long-term follow-up

What are the clinical outcomes of my protocols?

I have treated more than 600 hepatitis C patients. More than 80% have seen their conditions improve. Patients usually see their liver enzyme levels—especially ALT—improve or normalize in about two to three months. In the case of jaundice, the yellow color will be cleared up within two to three weeks. Subjective symptoms, such as fatigue, nausea, and poor appetite, improve within three to four weeks. Dull pain in the liver area ceases within a few weeks. After two or three months of taking herbs, a biopsy will show reduction of the inflammation. Many patients will see their viral load reduced and stabilized at a low level. I have also treated patients with cirrhosis who are already on a waiting list for liver transplant. Herbal treatments may be able to postpone liver transplant or improve the health of these patients in order to prepare them for a safer surgery. Their quality of life can also be improved.

What protocol did I use to achieve these clinical outcomes?

Based on Chinese studies, I have formulated my own protocol for treating chronic hepatitis C, as follows:

1. The use of anti-viral herbal remedies to reduce the viral load and suppress viral replication.

2. The use of liver-protective herbs to repair and heal damage caused by liver inflammation in order to normalize liver function.

3. The use of immune-regulating herbs to suppress auto-immune reactions, reduce production of circulatory immune complex, and strengthen immune function.

4. The use of blood-activating and stasis-expelling herbal formulas to improve the liver's microcirculation and promote liver cell regeneration and scar re-absorption.

5. The use of herbal formulas to facilitate bile secretion.

6. The treatment of hepatitis C-related clinical symptoms, such as fatigue, insomnia, joint pain, and skin rashes to improve quality of life.

How is the viral load lowered?

Suppressing the HCV viral load is achieved by strengthening immunity and using anti-viral herbal remedies. Immune regulation and enhancement will be discussed in a later section. Herbal treatment can reduce the viral load, but cannot totally eliminate it. Most herbal anti-viral studies have been conducted on HBV. The medicinal herbs *Polygoni cuspidati Rhizoma, Houttuyn Herbaiae, Rhei Rhizoma,* and *Blechni Rhizoma* have been found to suppress HBsAg in vitro. *Salviae miltiorrhziae Radix, Prunellae Spica, Gardeniae Fructus,* and *Moutan Radicis* have been found to suppress HBV-DNA polymerase activity more than 50% in vitro. HBV-DNAP is an important parameter to measure the replication of HBV. These herbs are common ingredients of formulas used for treating viral hepatitis. Clinically, when treated with these herbs, about 30 to 40% of patients' virus antigens—HBeAg, HBcAg, and HBsAg—turned to negative.

I have used the above-named herbs in a formula (HC Virostatic Formula), as well as olive leaf and its extract, to lower viral load. I have seen many of my patients' viral loads reduced and stabilized to below one million per milliliter.

I am conducting intensive research to develop more effective anti-HCV herbal remedies. Since anti-viral is the sole focus of conventional medicine, it has developed different anti-HCV treatment protocols. Severe side effects associated with these protocols are now limiting their use. The severity of the side effects is related to dosage. I believe that, if we can use smaller doses of these anti-viral drugs to avoid the side effects and combine them with herbal treatments to strengthen the anti-viral effects of the herbal treatments, together we might achieve better anti-viral efficacy.

How are liver enzyme levels normalized?

Normalizing liver enzyme levels and controlling inflammation are crucial factors in changing the poor prognosis of hepatitis C. Inflammation causes fibrosis (scarring), which leads to cirrhosis. Therefore, in order to halt the progression of chronic liver disease, controlling inflammation is crucial. If the liver is not actively inflamed, the median time for the development of cirrhosis is 80 years (Mathurin P. Moussalli et al., *Hepatology* 1998; 27:868-72). Since this is a near-normal life span, controlling inflammation is the main method to halt the progression of liver disease.

The active ingredients of *Schizandrae fructus*—schizandrin B and C—have been used in multiple-center clinical trials in China. In 4,558 cases, they were found to reduce ALT in 84-98% of the cases and normalize ALT in 75% of the cases within two to three months. We use these active ingredients with other herbs in our herbal formula Hepa Formula No. 2.

The active ingredient of *Ligustrum fructus*, oleanolic acid, has been used in a clinical study involving 153 patients, 110 cases (70%) of whom saw their ALT normalized within 50 days. A licorice root extract, glycyrrhizin, used to treat viral hepatitis in China and Japan showed a 64% (in Japan) and 85% (in China) efficacy rate for normalizing ALT. In my protocol, I use HEPA Formula No. 2, olenolic acid, and glycyrrhizin together and achieve a more than 80% rate of ALT improvement and more than 70% rate of normalization. For the non-responders (less than 20%), a second line of treatment has to be used.

How do we know the liver inflammation is under control?

The direct way to check liver inflammation is to do a biopsy. But a biopsy is invasive and carries the risk of morbidity. Most patients want to avoid it.

The indirect way to monitor inflammation is the ALT (SGPT) test. For untreated patients, this liver enzyme level in the blood fluctuates and is not closely related to liver inflammation. For treated patients, ALT is an important marker of liver inflammation. Following herbal treatment, most of our patients' ALT levels normalize. If tests show three consecutive normal readings and every reading is two to three months apart within one year's time, we can say that the liver inflammation is well under control. Besides liver function tests, clinical symptoms, such as liver area pain, fatigue, upper abdominal discomfort, nausea, and loose stool, should also diminish.

How can immunity be regulated?

HCV is a cytopathic and immunopathic virus. Most of the liver damage it causes is due to the body's inadequate immune response, especially auto-immune reactions. In the case of acute HCV infection, immune tolerance (insufficient reaction) causes the infection to become chronic. In chronic hepatitis, the over-active humeral immunity causes gamma-globulin levels to rise, which form the circulatory immune complex (CIC). When CIC deposits in the liver, joints, and skin, it causes inflammation. It is also the cause of cryoglobulinemia, a common complication of hepatitis C in which cold-sensitive globulin in the blood causes arthritis, skin rashes, and vasculitis. In cellular immunity, T suppresser cell function insufficiency and T helper cell hyperactivity make the inflammation persist.

In my protocol, I use the active ingredients of *Glycyrrhizae Radix* (licorice) and other herbs to suppress auto-immunity. These herbs also have anti-inflammatory effects. We use blood-activating and stasis-expelling herbs, the Circulation No. 1 Tablet, to clear the CIC. I use the following herbs to regulate cellular immunity: *Cordyceps sinensis, Sophorae subprostratae Radix,* and *Polyporus umbellatus Pers.*

I have seen very positive responses to immune-regulatory treatments. Strengthened immunity is the major force that our bodies use to fight off the virus. Immune regulation is a complicated task. Much study needs to be done to improve the immune-regulatory effects of herbal medicine.

Why is facilitation of bile secretion important?

The bile of patients with chronic viral hepatitis is usually thick and blocked by inflamed liver tissue. This can cause jaundice, gallbladder inflammation, and gallstones. Bile retention can further injure the liver and promote fibrosis. In blood tests, bile retention shows up as elevated GGT, AKP, and bilirubin levels. Therefore, facilitating bile secretion is very important. The Gall No. 1 Formula, which consists of *Artemisiae capillaris Herba, Bupleuri Radix, Desmodii Herba, Taraxaci Herba, Isatidis Radix, Lonicerae Flos,* and *Gentianae scabrae Radix,* can effectively release bile retention and eliminate jaundice in a few weeks. Symptoms such as nausea, dark urine, and pale stool can be relieved in about a month. This formula can also be used for gallbladder inflammation and gallstones.

What can be done to improve microcirculation?

Studies conducted at Chinese research hospitals revealed that chronic viral hepatitis patients have obvious blood circulation disorders, especially microcirculation disorders. In Chinese medicine, this condition is called blood stagnancy. Typically, patients have liver palms, spider moles, cold hands and feet, purplish tongue, dark lips, dark rings around the eyes, and enlarged spleen. Use of a blood-activating and stasis-expelling herbal formula, such as Circulation No. 1 Tablets (a modification of Persica & Achyranthes Combination), can improve these symptoms. With improvement of microcirculation in the liver comes liver-cell regeneration and suppression of hypertrophy of the interstitial connective tissue, thus preventing fibrosis.

How can cirrhosis be prevented?

If no proper treatment is given, about 25% of patients with chronic hepatitis will develop cirrhosis in 20 to 30 years. If the liver disease is properly treated and the inflammation controlled, even though the HCV is still present, the median time for the development of cirrhosis is about 80 years. In short, controlling liver inflammation is the first step in preventing cirrhosis. The second step is to facilitate bile secretion, the third is to improve microcirculation, and the fourth is to remove the CIC and regulate immunity.

In China, herbs used for silicosis (miner's lung) to suppress the fibroblastic activities have been used for treating early-stage cirrhosis. Controlled animal studies found that in cirrhotic animal models treated with these herbs, liver collagen content was much lower than in the untreated control group.

Cordyceps sinensis, Persicae Semen, Salvia miltiorrhizae, Glycyrrhizin, and *Aristolochiae fangchi Radix* can decompose collagen and soften the liver, while at the same time promote liver-cell regeneration.

What constitutes a cure for hepatitis C?

"Cure" is a strong word, and different medical systems have their own definitions. Chinese medicine defines "cure" as the body's return to balance and normal functioning. Western medicine, on the other hand, focuses on the disease-causing agent, HCV, and its definition, therefore, is the complete elimination of the virus. The differences between these two definitions have led to different emphases in treatment strategies and different protocols. Both TCM and Western practitioners need to be aware that establishing unreachable goals can frustrate both the patient and the practitioner.

In health care, the ultimate aim of treatment is to restore a person's health and normal life expectancy. Eliminating the virus is one method of reaching this aim. Philosophically speaking, the method should serve the aim and not vice versa. We must not attempt to eliminate the HCV at any cost, even at the cost of the patient's health. Rebetron treatment may temporarily cause about half of the patients to lower their HCV load and improve their liver function tests. But along with these improvements is the deterioration of quality of life. Many patients become sicker and weaker while their lab markers improve.

Chinese medical treatments may not be able to reduce the HCV load to the levels that conventional anti-viral treatment can; they can only lower the HCV load and stabilize it. But TCM can definitely help the majority of patients lower or normalize their liver enzyme levels and halt disease progression. Although long-term treatment may be required, quality of life is definitely improved. We know that when the liver inflammation is well under control, cirrhosis takes a long time to develop.

The realistic aim of Chinese medical treatment for hepatitis C is the arrest and reversal of HCV-related problems, resulting in improved or normal function and a reasonable expectation of an average life span.

One of my patient's stories illustrates this realistic approach. Joseph V is a New Jersey firefighter, diagnosed with hepatitis C in 1996. When he came to our clinic, he was on disability, and his liver enzyme levels were above 300 (normal is below 40). He felt tired all the time and could not work or go to the gym. He came to see me in 1997. After two months of treatment with herbal remedies, his liver enzyme levels normalized and he went back to firefighting. Later, his conventional doctor convinced him to try alpha interferon and he didn't want to lose the chance to try this FDA-approved therapy. He stopped herbal treatments and went on alpha interferon for eight months. During that time, he returned to disability and felt very sick. When the treatment course finished, his liver enzyme levels had shot up to 380. At that point, his conventional doctor suggested that he add ribavarin to alpha interferon. He said he had had enough and refused. He came back to see me and resumed the herbal treatment. Within two months, his liver function normalized again. He went back to firefighting and got married. He told me that before the herbal treatment, he had lost his confidence and had no long-term life plan. The herbal treatment helped him put his life together again and gave him the confidence to start a family. Since resuming herbal treatment, he has furthered his education and been promoted to captain.

"Pure water has no fish."

Many patients worry that they are carrying a virus and have not been cured. Although their liver functions are normalized and they have a normal or near-normal quality of life, they feel uneasy that they still have HCV in their body. I tell them that everybody carries certain viruses in his or her body. It is abnormal not to have viruses in our bodies. Some viruses have names and can be tested; some have no names and can't be tested. Viruses were the first living things on Earth and are one of the major causes of mutation. Bad mutations die off and good mutations become higher living things. We human beings are the highest living things on Earth—thanks to the virus. In millions of years of evolution, the human body has adopted mechanisms to deal with viruses. Given enough time, it will learn how to coexist with a newly invading virus. Gradually, our immune system can control it, keep it at bay, and prevent it from further harm.

No living things are pure. There is a Chinese saying: "Pure water has no fish." Why do we want our bodies to be so pure, without viruses? Worrying can only weaken the immune system and make the virus stronger. From the experiences of many of our HIV patients, we have seen that coexistence with the virus is possible. After coexisting for a sufficiently long time, the virus becomes less harmful and finally becomes harmless, while at same time our body becomes stronger and can contain the virus better.

Conclusion

Although Chinese herbal treatments may not be a cure for chronic liver diseases—at least according to the conventional medical definition—they present alternatives for hepatitis C patients. What's more, they have no serious side effects. They can definitely improve overall health and halt the progress of chronic hepatitis. At least these herbal treatments enable us to buy more time for patients to wait for new treatment discoveries in the future. Furthermore, TCM herbal treatment is much less expensive than conventional therapies. For chronic hepatitis, the sooner herbal treatment is given, the better the results.

2

Chinese Herbal Therapeutics for Hepatitis C

In this chapter, clinical treatment of hepatitis C will be discussed: which herbal formulas to use; when and how to use them; adverse reactions; how long to use the herbs; and how to monitor the efficacy of herbal treatment. Treatments for some hepatitis C-related symptoms and complications will be discussed in Chapter 3.

Chronic viral hepatitis, especially hepatitis C, is a complicated liver disease. Liver damage is mainly caused by inadequate immune response. HCV replication alone causes little direct damage. Simply eliminating HCV is insufficient to heal the damage already done by the chronic disease over 20 to 30 years. Effective treatment should address both pathogenetic and etiologic problems. My Chinese herbal treatment protocol for hepatitis C is just such a comprehensive and systematic approach. It consists of eight treatment objectives:

1. Control of liver inflammation and normalization of liver function, i.e., lowering or normalizing ALT level.

2. Lowering and stabilizating of the viral load at a low level (below one million per milliliter) or eradication of the HCV.

3. Regulation of immunity to help achieve the two above-mentioned goals.

4. Improvement of microcirculation in the liver in order to promote liver regeneration.

5. Facilitating bile secretion and excretion.

6. Lowering portal vein pressure, and prevention and reversal of fibrosis.

7. Maintenance of normalized liver function and halting liver-disease progression (after liver inflammation is well under control).

8. Treatment of hepatitis C-related symptoms and complications, such as fatigue, insomnia, joint pain, skin rashes, diabetes, and infections, thus improving the patient's overall health.

Treatment consists of herbs used singly and in formulas. The ingredients and their phytopharmacological actions are discussed in Chapter 4.

1. Control of liver inflammation and normalization of liver function

This requires the improvement and normalization of enzyme levels and the healing of inflamed liver cells. The herbal remedies listed below are necessary for most patients, especially those with elevated ALT and AST levels. These enzymes are normally found inside the liver cells, though they leak into the bloodstream when liver cells are inflamed. This is especially true of ALT, which exists mostly in liver cells and has more specificity for monitoring liver inflammation than AST does.

Moreover, ALT responds to herbal treatment much faster than AST. AST exists in the heart and muscle, as well as the liver, and is less specific to liver inflammation and responds to treatment more slowly than ALT does. In order to control liver inflammation, three consecutive normal ALT readings within one year must be seen, and each reading should be two to three months apart. Hence, this part of treatment should last at least one year. This group of herbal remedies can also help maintain normal enzyme levels for those patients with a normal ALT level.

Hepa Formula No. 2 Capsule

Each capsule contains 500mg extracts of the formula. Dose: 2 capsules, 3 times a day, 10 to 20 minutes before each meal.

Ligustrin Capsule

Each capsule contains 40mg oleaolic acid and other herbal extracts. Dose: 1 capsule, 3 times a day, 10 to 20 minutes before each meal.

Glycyrrhizin Capsule

Each capsule contains 150mg of glycyrrhizin and other herbal extracts. Dose: 1 capsule, 2 times a day, 10 to 20 minutes before each meal.

Caution: About 20% of patients taking Glycyrrhizin Capsule may experience headache and elevated blood pressure. This capsule is contra-indicated for patients with hypertension. If blood pressure rises, the herb should be discontinued. Blood pressure will normalize after discontinuing use of this herb. Since Glycyrrhizin Capsule can deplete potassium in the body, patients should consume potassium-rich bananas and potassium supplement (93 mg per day) while taking Glycyrrhizin Capsules.

Circulation Tablet No. 1

Each tablet contains 500mg of formula extracts.
Dose: 4 tablets, 3 times a day, taken with a meal.

The above formulas are the first line of herbal remedies for improving and normalizing liver function. To facilitate ordering these herbal products, we have placed them into two groups: Group I includes all four herbal products, Group II contains all but Glycyrrhizin Capsule. Group II is for those who have high blood pressure.

As a result of taking these herbs, most (80%) patients' liver function will improve or normalize within two to three months. After taking these herbs for two to three months, liver function tests should be repeated. After these tests show normal readings, it is important to continue taking these herbs in order to have three consecutive normal readings within one year.

If a patient does not respond to these herbs, a second line of herbal remedies should be used. Patients should consult with me on an individual basis regarding this protocol.

2. Lowering and stabilization of the viral load or eradication of the HCV

Because hepatitis C is an infectious disease, it is important to completely eliminate or at least lower the HCV load, especially for those with a high (greater than one million per milliliter) HCV load. To suppress HCV replication we rely mainly on the body's own immunity. Herbal treatment can help to strengthen immune response. Patients can use the following herbal products to lower their HCV load.

HC Virostatic Capsule

Each capsule contains 500mg of formula extracts. Dose: 2 capsules, 3 times a day, 10 to 20 minutes before each meal.

Glycyrrhizin Capsule (see #1 above)

Olive Leaf Decoction

Decoction made from olive leaves is made by soaking a half pound of olive leaves in one gallon of water. Simmer at 175° F for 12 hours in a crock pot. Strain the leaves out of the decoction, and keep liquid in the refrigerator. Drink 3 ounces, 2 times a day.

Olive Leaf Extract, Olivessence Capsule

Dose: 1 capsule, 2 times a day.

These herbal remedies can reduce the viral load. Most of my patients take only one or two products from this category. The viral load will fluctuate with mental and physical stresses, but by using these herbal remedies, the viral load can be lowered and stabilized for most patients.

3. Regulation of immunity

HCV causes cytopathic and immunopathic damage to the liver. Immunopathology is the main pathology in chronic hepatitis. It causes globulinemia, cryoglobulinemia, rashes, joint pain and swelling, and many hepatitis-related autoimmune complications, such as diabetes, thyroid gland inflammation, Sjögren's syndrome, psoriasis, arthritis, and vasculitis. Regulating immunity includes suppressing overactive humeral immunity (reducing anti-body production, especially auto-antibody production), promoting CD8 cell function, and removing the circulatory immune complex (CIC) deposition in the liver, skin, and joints. Regulating immunity is an important precondition of normalizing liver function and lowering the HCV load. Suppressing auto-immunity is especially important for chronic active hepatitis.

Glycyrrhizin Capsule (see #1 above)

AI Capsule No. 3

Each capsule contains 100mg of extracts of *Mucunae Caulis*, *Sargentodoxae cuneata Caulis*, and *Paederiae Caulis*. Dose: 1 capsule, 3 times a day, with food.

Circulation Tablet No. 1 (see # 1 above)

Cordyceps Capsule

Each capsule contains 300mg extract of *Cordyceps sinensis hyphas mycelium*. Dose: 2 capsules, 3 times a day, 10 to 20 minutes before meals.

With this treatment, we can see obvious improvement in the symptoms and signs of autoimmune reactions. Immune regulation is a very complex treatment and we still do not thoroughly understand the detailed immunological changes during the course of viral hepatitis. Much research is needed for further improvement of this treatment.

4. Improvement of microcirculation in the liver in order to promote liver regeneration

Improving microcirculation and blood rheology is an important part of this treatment protocol. The majority of patients with chronic liver disease have blood circulation—especially microcirculation—disorders. In TCM, this is known as blood stagnancy. When microcirculation deteriorates, liver tissue does not receive proper nutrition and oxygen, which leads to fibrosis (scar formation). Improving microcirculation can prevent fibrosis and promote liver-cell regeneration.

Circulation Tablet No. 1 (see #1 above)

5. Facilitating bile secretion and excretion

Bile retention can injure the liver, promote fibrosis, and cause jaundice. In blood tests, it causes a rise in GGT, AKP (alkaline phosphatese), and bilirubin levels. Therefore, facilitating bile secretion is very important. About 50% of chronic hepatitis patients have gallstones and chronic gallbladder inflammation. I prescribe the following herbal formulas to facilitate the secretion and excretion of gall juice and to control gallbladder inflammation:

Gall Formula No. 1

> Each tablet contains 500mg of the formula extract. Dose: 3 tablets, 3 times a day, 10 to 20 minutes before meals.

Capillaris Combination Capsule

> Each capsule contains 500mg of the formula extract. Dose: 4 capsules, 3 times a day, 10 to 20 minutes before meals, or

Capillaris Combination Granule

> A bottle contains 100g of granulated formula. Dose: 2g, 3 times a day, 10 to 20 minutes before meals.

6. Lowering portal vein pressure and prevention and reversal of fibrosis

When liver disease is advanced, one common complication is portal vein hypertension (high blood pressure in the portal vein), a condition that can cause ascites (water in the stomach), enlarged spleen, varices in the esophagus and stomach, hemorrhoids, and bleeding. A very important objective in the treatment of advanced cases of chronic liver disease is the lowering of portal vein pressure.

Red Peony Combination Capsule

Each capsule contains 500mg of the formula extracts. Dose: 4 capsules, 3 times a day, 10 to 20 minutes before meals, or

Red Peony Combination Granule

A bottle contains 100g of granulated formula. Dose: 2g, 3 times a day, 10 to 20 minutes before meals.

Red Peony Combination has a special effect of lowering portal vein pressure and is an important treatment in advanced hepatitis and in early stages of cirrhosis.

Circulation Tablet No. 1 (see #1 above)

Circulation Tablet No. 1 can improve oxygen and nutrition supply to inflamed liver tissue, which will reduce overgrowth of the interstitial connective tissue and thus reduce fibrosis.

Cordyceps Capsule (see #3 above)

Glycyrrhizin Capsule (see #1 above)

Cordyceps and glycyrrhizin have been shown to have inhibitory effects on fibrosis in animal models of cirrhosis.

7. Maintenance of normalized liver function and the halting of liver-disease progression

We can use the maintenance protocol only after three consecutive normal ALT readings within one year, with readings taken two to three months apart, and disappearance of most subjective clinical symptoms. Test results of AST, GGT, AKP, and bilirubin must also be normal or near-normal. This protocol has to be used on a long-term basis. The herbs in this protocol have no adverse reactions and virtually no toxicity, therefore, they can be used indefinitely. They can be considered daily supplements, like vitamins. Long-term use of these herbs can help maintain normal liver function and enhance general health.

Hepa Formula No. 3

Hepa Formula No. 3 is for those patients with normalized ALT and other enzymes, but with fibrosis staging greater than stage 2 (S2). This formula maintains normal liver enzyme levels and has anti-fibrosis effects. Each bottle contains 100g of the granulated formula. Dose: 2g, 3 times a day, 10 to 20 minutes before meals.

Hepa Formula No. 4 Capsule

Each capsule contains 500mg of the formula extracts. Dose: 2 capsules, 3 times a day, 10 to 20 minutes before meals.

Circulation Tablet No. 4

Each tablet contains 500mg of the formula extracts. Dose: 2 tablets, 3 times a day, with food.

Cordyceps Capsule (see #3 above)

8. Treatment of hepatitis C-related symptoms and complications

This will be discussed in Chapter 3.

3

Clinical Therapeutics for Hepatitis C-Related Conditions

In this chapter, herbal treatments for hepatitis C-related symptoms and complications, such as fatigue, insomnia, joint pain, skin rashes, vasculitis, psoriasis, Sjögren's syndrome, diabetes, infections, ascites and edema, bleeding, and nausea and vomiting, will be discussed. The ingredients and pharmacological actions of these formulas and single herbs can be found in Chapter 4.

Fatigue

The liver is the major powerhouse of the body. Most of our energy supply for daily activities comes from the liver. Once liver function deteriorates, we naturally will feel fatigued—the primary complaint of chronic hepatitis patients. Treating fatigue relies mainly on the improvement of liver function. If fatigue is the major problem and isn't relieved after liver function is normalized, Cordyceps Capsule is prescribed.

● Cordyceps Capsule (see Chapter 2)

Insomnia

Insomnia is a common complaint of chronic viral hepatitis patients. Conventional sleeping aids are usually addictive and hard on the liver. An alternative sleeping aid without side effects is needed, since it is crucial that the body have adequate sleep to aid the healing process.

- HerbSom Capsule
  Each capsule contains 300mg of the formula extracts.
  Dose: 2 capsules at bedtime.

It is the best sleeping aid in Chinese medicine, as it is not addictive and does not induce daytime drowsiness. Most importantly for hepatitis patients, it does not harm the liver.

Joint Pain, Skin Rashes, Vasculitis, Psoriasis, and Sjögren's Syndrome

In addition to these symptoms and complications, some hepatitis patients also have positive reactions to ANA, AMA, and RA factors. These extra-liver manifestations of immunopathic damages (autoimmunity) caused by HCV infections have a common pathological mechanism; hence the treatment is similar.

- AI Capsule No. 3 (see Chapter 2)
- Circulation Tablet No. 1 (see Chapter 2)

Diabetes

One of the liver's functions is regulating blood sugar. Following a meal, the blood sugar level increases. This sugar turns into glycogen and is stored in the liver. When the blood sugar level decreases, liver glycogen is decomposed into glucose and released into the bloodstream to maintain a normal blood sugar level. With chronic hepatitis, this function deteriorates and many patients see their blood sugar levels rise. HCV causes autoimmune reactions that can also damage the beta cells of the pancreas and affect insulin production. Both factors can cause hepatitis C-related diabetes.

● BM Capsule (Bitter Melon)
Each capsule contains 500mg of the formula extract. Dose: 3 capsules, 3 times a day, 10 to 20 minutes before meals.

Infections

Occasionally, in the course of chronic hepatitis C, patients will contract infections, such as sore throat, sinusitis, common cold, and bronchitis. To fight off these infections, physicians prescribe antibiotics, some of which may harm the liver. Chinese medicine avoids harmful antibiotics and instead uses herbal remedies, including the high-potency garlic extract allicin. Garlic has become very popular, but most garlic products sold in health food stores are odorless and therefore pharmacologically useless in fighting infections. The garlic odor carried by allicin is the very substance that has anti-infectious effects. The garlic products used in my clinic are all composed of pharmacologically active allicin. The allicin we use for our patients is 4,000 to 6,000 times more potent than the odorless garlic sold in health food stores. In addition, Coptin and Rhubarbin tablets may also be used to fight infections.

● Time Release Allicin Capsule
Each capsule contains 20mg of allicin. Dose: for preventive use, 1 capsule per day; for treating acute infections, 2 or 3 capsules, 3 times a day.

- Allicin Vial

  Each vial contains 30mg of allicin in 2 ml of solution. Dose: 1 vial diluted in 8 ounces water, once or twice a day.

- Coptin Tablet

  Each tablet contains 100mg of coptin, an extract of *Coptis Rhizoma*. Dose: 2 tablets, 3 times a day, 10 to 20 minutes before meals.

- Rhubarbin Tablet

  Each tablet contains 500mg of rhubarbin, an extract of *Rhei Rhizoma* (rhubarb root). Dose: 2 tablets, 3 times a day, or follow health practitioner's advice.

Ascites and Edema

Ascites and edema generally occur when liver disease has advanced to cirrhosis. They are caused by hypertension in the portal vein and low albumin in the serum, which decrease osmotic pressure of the blood. Ascites usually accompanies lower leg or ankle swelling. If these symptoms occur, the patient should limit salt intake. Concurrently, an herbal formula can be used to expel the water.

- Stephania & Astragalus Combination

  Dose: 4 capsules, 3 times a day, or 2g of the granulated formula, 3 times a day, 10 to 20 minutes before meals.

Bleeding

Bleeding becomes a problem when liver disease advances to the cirrhosis stage, especially when portal vein pressure increases and varices form in the stomach and esophagus. At this stage, blood-clotting factors produced by the liver decrease and platelet counts are depleted. All these risk factors make bleeding a serious problem. Dangerously severe bleeding, such as black stool or bloody vomiting, can cause blood pressure to drop dramatically. Though rare, once this happens, the patient should be rushed to an emergency room. More common is gum bleeding during teeth brushing and nose bleeding. For these conditions, the following herbal capsule is used.

● Yunnan Pai Yao Capsule
Dose: 1 capsule, 4 times a day, 10 to 20 minutes before meals and before bed.

Diarrhea

Diarrhea is a common complaint of chronic hepatitis patients. Most diarrhea improves as liver function improves. If this symptom persists and/or becomes severe, treatment is required.

● Ginseng & Atractylodes Formula
Dose: 4 capsules, 3 times a day; or 2g of the granulated formula, 3 times a day, 10 to 20 minutes before meals.

Nausea and Vomiting

Nausea is more common than vomiting, especially when bile secretion is blocked and digestion is affected. Usually, these symptoms improve as liver function improves. If these complaints become persistent and intolerable, they can be treated with the following herbal formula.

● Pinellia & Hoelen Combination
Dose: 4 capsules, 3 times a day, or 2g of granulated formula, 3 times a day, 10 to 20 minutes before meals.

4

Herbal Remedies and Their Pharmacology

The herbal remedies I use to treat viral hepatitis consist of single herbs and formulas. All are made from herbal extracts and active ingredients, the phytochemistry and pharmacology of which have been well studied. Clinical applications are based on their pharmacology and traditional usage in TCM. With the development of new extraction and purification techniques, we can now use more potent forms of the herbal remedies and, hence, smaller doses. Therapeutic actions are predictable and can be replicated. In this section I discuss their pharmacology and main usage in TCM as pertains to the treatment of viral hepatitis.

The most common criticism of herbal medicine is that herbs are not stable in respect to their active essence, since species, collecting seasons, and production sites vary. Furthermore, the method of preparation (drying, steaming, and decocting) may dilute the active essence of the herb. It is also argued that herbal medicines are inconvenient to prepare for ingestion. Finally, herbal medicines are often bitter and unpleasant to ingest. These drawbacks can be mitigated through scientific preparation procedures to achieve a consistent pharmacological effect. What's more, extracts can be concentrated to the point that the daily dosage is small and requires no special preparation. And since capsule, tablet, and granular forms of herbal preparations are placed on the tongue and swallowed with a large glass of water, poor taste is no longer a deterrent.

I am fully aware that herbal products are not strictly regulated, and therefore am very careful in choosing my supply. I check whether the manufacturer exerts an acceptable level of control over the nature and quality of the raw materials and the procedures followed in their processing. The manufacturer I use follows GMP (Good Manufacture Practice) standards, and the formulas and single herbal products I use contain highly purified active ingredients.

HERBAL FORMULAS

Over centuries of clinical experience, TCM doctors have learned to compound herbal formulas on the basis of the properties and flavors of individual herbs used to treat specific diseases. These formulas are usually composed of 8 to 12 herbs. Most TCM formulas are made from a combination of four types of herbs:

* the emperor herb(s),

* the minister herb(s),

* the assistant herb(s), and

* the servant herb(s).

Emperor and minister herbs are synergistic and perform major pharmacological actions. Assistant herbs counterbalance possible side effects of the emperor and minister herbs. Servant herbs direct the actions of the other herbs to their target organs. The formulas discussed in this section are organized according to this principle and their pharmacological actions.

Hepa Formula No. 2

A. Herbal Composition

Schizandrae Fructus, Artemisiae capillaris Herba, Alismatis Rhizoma, Polyporus, Poria (hoelen), *Atractylodes Rhizoma, Cinnamomi Ramulus, Citri Pericarpium, Magnoliae Cortex, Zingiberis Rhizoma* (ginger), and *Glycyrrhizae Radix* (licorice)

B. Pharmacology of Major Ingredients

Schizandrae Fructus is the major ingredient. The pharmacological effects of its active ingredients have been studied extensively.

Animal studies have shown that alcohol extracts of the kernel of the fruit of schizandra (AEKFS) have many pharmacological activities such as:

1. Lowering the ALT elevation caused by carbon tetrachloride (CCl_4)-induced liver damage.

2. Reducing CCl_4-induced fat deposits in liver cells.

3. Reducing CCl_4-induced histological damage of liver cells.

4. Promoting glycogen and serum protein synthesis in the liver.

5. Promoting regeneration after partial removal of the liver.

6. Increasing metabolic enzymes in the liver.

Clinical trials using tablets made from AEKFS, conducted in three hospitals in China, found that in 107 chronic viral hepatitis cases, 73 cases' ALT levels normalized and clinical symptoms improved following treatment with *Schizandrae Fructus*. No serious side effects were reported.

From the fruit of schizandra, seven active liver-enzyme-lowering ingredients have been isolated. Schizandrin B and C can enhance the detoxification function of the liver and promote protein and liver glycogen synthesis. A precursor of synthesized schizandrin C can effectively normalize liver function. The effectiveness rate of schizandrins in lowering liver enzymes is around 80%. The enzyme level may rebound in about 60% of the patients a half month to six months after treatment is stopped. Clinical observation found that schizandra was better in lowering ALT than AST and has no effect in turning HBsAg to negative.

Schizandra can improve the function of the liver cell membrane and reduce its leakage. Animal studies found that extract of schizandra can suppress the activity of ALT, but there was no effect on AST or LDH.

At the Sixth National Hepatitis Conference of China (1990), it was reported that in the carbon tetrachloride toxic model of human liver embryo cell culture, extracts of schizandra significantly reduced cell damage and kept cell membranes intact. The report concluded that schizandra can protect the liver cell membrane.

The pharmacological actions of *Artemisiae capillaris Herba*, *Glycyrrhizae Radix*, and *Polyporus* are discussed below in regards to other herbal formulas and single herbs.

C. Clinical Use

Hepa Formula No. 2 is used clinically to lower and normalize ALT and other liver enzyme levels. In my clinic, it is the primary treatment for the control of liver inflammation.

D. Package

One bottle of Hepa Formula No. 2 contains 180 capsules, enough for 1 month.

E. Dose

Take 2 capsules, 3 times a day, 10 to 20 minutes before meals.

Hepa Formula No. 3

A. Herbal Composition

Schizandrae Fructus, Artemisiae capillaris Herba, Polyporus, Poria (hoelen), *Atractylodes Rhizoma, Cinnamomi Ramulus, Zingiberis Rhizoma* (ginger), *Glycyrrhizae Radix* (licorice), *Persicae Semen, Salviae miltiorrhizae Radix, Zedoariae Rhizoma,* and *Sparganii Rhizoma*

The basic composition of this formula is the same as Hepa Formula No. 2, though herbs to improve microcirculation and prevent fibrosis have been added.

B. Pharmacology of Major Ingredients

Schizandrae Fructus is the major ingredient. Its pharmacology is discussed in the previous formula.

Salviae miltiorrhizae Radix (salvia) is the main added ingredient. It markedly improves microcirculation and prevents fibrosis. In TCM, it is used for activating blood circulation to dispel blood stasis, clearing heart fire to ease anxiety and cool the blood, and dispelling accumulation (tumor).

The pharmacological actions of salvia that pertain to liver disease:

1. Salvia improves microcirculation in the liver. Measuring the blood flow in acute and chronic CCl_4

toxic models of rats found that salvia treatment can markedly increase blood flow in the liver. Liver-protective and fibrosis-preventive effects of salvia are mainly the result of its effects in improving microcirculation.

2. Salvia improves microcirculation in coronary heart patients, 70% of whom saw their conjunctival and nailfold microcirculation improve. In animal studies, salvia extract reversed peripheral microcirculation blockage caused by intravenous infusion of 10% dextran. Salvia can increase blood supply to the heart and ischemic tissue.

3. Salvia protects liver cells. In the CCl_4 acute toxic rat model, salvia quickly lowered ALT and reduced in-flammatory reactions such as cytonecrosis (cell death) and steatosis (fat degeneration). In the chronic CCl_4 toxic animal model, salvia extract lowered ALT and reduced collagen formation. In the control group, CCl_4 caused collagen and globulin to increase from 19.8mg/g to 51.4mg/g and 14.21mg/g to 23.04mg/g in liver tissue, respectively. Moreover, every rat in the control group developed cirrhosis. In the salvia-treated group, not a single rat developed cirrhosis, nor did collagen and globulin increase. This shows that salvia not only suppresses fibrosis formation but can also reverse existing fibrosis.

C. Clinical Use

This formula maintains lowered and normalized ALT and prevents fibrosis.

D. Package

One bottle contains 100g of the granulated formula.

E. Dose

Take 2g, 3 times a day, with water, 10 to 20 minutes before meals.

Hepa Formula No. 4

After the liver enzyme level has been normalized, the patient needs a long-term maintenance formula to keep liver function normal.

A. Herbal Composition

Schizandrae Fructus, Ligustri Fructus, Glycyrrhizae Radix (licorice), *Sophorae subprostratae Radix, Salviae miltiorrhizae Radix, Paeoniae rubra Radix,* and *Cnidii Rhizoma*

B. Pharmacology of Major Ingredients

Schizandrae Fructus and *Salviae miltiorrhizae Radix* are the major ingredients. Their pharmacology has been discussed previously.

The pharmacological effects of *Ligustri Fructus* and *Glycyrrhizae Radix* (licorice) will be discussed later in the single-herbs section.

The active ingredient of *Sophorae subprostratae Radix* is oxymatrine. In three commonly used liver-damage models (CCl$_4$-induced rabbit, rat, and mouse), oxymatrine prevented liver-cell damage. Compared with the control group, the oxymatine-treated group had much lower ALT, less liver-cell necrosis, and much less inflammation. Oxymatrine increases cell pigment P-450 content and activity and increases smooth-surfaced endoplasmic reticulum of the liver cell. It is an inducer of cytochrome P-450, thus it can strengthen the detoxification capability of the liver. Recently, it has shown anti-viral effects. Its anti-inflammatory, immune-regulatory, anti-cancer, and leukogenic (raising white blood cell count) effects are also useful in treating viral hepatitis.

C. Clinical Use

Hepa Formula No. 4 is for long-term maintenance, since it keeps the ALT level stable.

D. Package

Each capsule contains 500mg of the formula extracts. One bottle contains 180 capsules, enough for 1 month.

E. Dose

Take 2 capsules, 3 times a day, 10 to 20 minutes before meals.

Gall Formula No. 1

A. Herbal Composition

Bupleuri Radix, Artemisiae capillaris Herba, Desmodii Herba, Taraxaci Herba, Gardeniae Fructus, Saussureae Radix, Citri Pericarpium, Citri immaturi Pericarpium, Salviae miltiorrhizae Radix, Angelica Radix, Scutellariae Radix, and *Gentianae Radix*

B. Pharmacology of Major Ingredients

Bupleuri Radix is well-known in TCM for its liver-protective and cholagogic (facilitating bile secretion) actions. It can protect the liver from toxic damage caused by galactosamine. It also can protect the liver from injury due to CCl_4 and the mold *Penicillium notatum*. In animal studies, it has been shown to increase bile secretion and the amount of bile salt contained in the bile. It is a choleretic (stimulating secretion of bile) substance and can normalize the bile-secreting function of the liver and normalize the chemical composition of the bile (the proportion of bilirubin and cholesterol). Its anti-inflammatory effect can be used for cholangitis (inflammation of the gallbladder).

Artemisiae capillaris Herba, the main TCM herb for jaundice, has the following pharmacological actions:

1. Capillaris promotes bile secretion and excretion. It possesses cholagogic effects on both healthy animals and those with CCl_4-induced liver damage.

   One of the choleretic and cholagogic constituents of capillaris is 6,7-dimethoxycoumarin, infusion of which at 0.2 and 0.3 g/kg into the duodenum of anesthetized rats increased bile secretion 0.5 hour later by a mean of 50% and 180%, respectively. In dogs with chronic gallbladder fistulae, administration of 6,7-dimethoxycourmarin at 0.3g/kg by mouth increased the production of bile by a mean of 74% in 3 hours. In rats, the use of this agent in combination with genipin obtained from the fruit of *Gardeniae jasminoides* produced a synergistic effect in promoting bile secretion. Its decoction can decrease the tone of the Oddi's sphincter in anesthetized dogs.

   Two other cholertic and cholgogic principles, capillarisin and methylcapillarisin, have been isolated from capillaris and have proved to be more potent than 6,7-dimethoxycoumarin.

2. Capillaris protects the liver. After daily injection of its decoction—0.61g to rats with CCl_4-induced liver damage—histological examination on the 8th day revealed that swelling of liver cells, fatty degeneration, and necrosis were mild, compared with the

control group. Liver glycogen and RNA content
were normalized or almost recovered, and ALT activity was markedly reduced. This evidence suggests
that the herb possesses a liver-protective action.

3. Capillaris' anti-lipemic (lowering blood lipids) and
   fibrolytic effects are applicable to chronic viral
   hepatitis treatment. Clinically, it has been used for
   hepatitis, biliary tract infections, and cholelithiasis
   (gallstones).

Desmodii styracifolium Herba is the main herb of Lithagogic
Decoction for gallstones, since it possesses cholagogic,
choleretic (facilitating bile secretion), and lithogogic (expelling
gallstones) effects. Intravenous infusion into the femoral vein
or intraduodenal administration of the decoction of this herb
at 8g/kg to dogs can markedly increase the bile collected.
Drainage of the human duodenum showed that it had a
choleretic action. Bile excretion is probably promoted by the
relaxation of the Oddi's sphincter following increase of intraductal pressure consequent to increase of bile secreted by
liver cells. Choleretic action facilitates excretion of sandy
stones, abates biliary obstruction and pain, and causes subsidence of jaundice.

In both acute and chronic experiments, bile flow from the
gallbladder was greatly increased in dogs given Lithagogic
Decoction in which *Desmodii* is the chief ingredient. Furthermore, bile secretion was increased by 3 to 20 times, and solid
components in the bile were markedly decreased in 6 out of 7
anesthetized dogs, 10 to 20 minutes after administration of
Lithagogic Decoction. Simultaneously, the Oddi's sphincter
relaxed, coinciding with peak choleretic effect. A 20-60% in-

crease in bile secretion associated with relaxation of the Oddi's sphincter in 4 cases of biliary fistulae was achieved after administration of this decoction. In vitro studies using fresh bile obtained from patients suffering from bile pigment stones showed that Lithagogic Decoction prevented the precipitation of stone-forming elements, indicating that this herb has an anti-lithiasis (stone-forming) effect. The action of Lithagogic Decoction was said to be related to the inhibition of beta-glucuronidase activity in the bile. The decoction appeared to minimize the formation of new stones in rabbits with transplanted cholesterol gallstones. It has been used clinically for gallbladder inflammation and stones.

The pharmacology of *Salviae miltiorrhizae Radix* was previously discussed.

C. Clinical Use

Gall Formula No. 1 facilitates secretion of bile and heals inflammation in the gallbladder. It can also help in flushing out sand-like calculi (sandy stones) and help lower and normalize GGT, AKP, and bilirubin, total and direct. Gall Formula No. 1 should be used if the patient shows signs of jaundice and bile retention (yellowish skin and conjunctiva, dark urine, pale stool, and itchy skin).

D. Package

Each tablet contains 500mg of formula extracts. One bottle contains 270 tablets, enough for 1 month.

E. Dose

Take 3 tablets, 3 times a day, 10 to 20 minutes before meals.

HC Virostatic Formula

HC Virostatic Formula suppresses HCV replication and lowers viral load, making it an important treatment in my hepatitis C protocol.

A. Herbal Composition

Sophorae subprostratae Radix, Polygoni cuspidati Rhizoma, Rhei Rhizoma, Baphicacanthis Folium, Isatidis Radix, and *Houttuyniae Herba*

B. Pharmacology of Major Ingredients

The active ingredient of *Sophorae subprostratae Radix* is oxymatrine, and its pharmacological actions are discussed above (see Hepa Formula No. 4).

Polygoni cuspidati Rhizoma has anti-viral effects. A 10% decoction of this herb inhibited Asian influenza virus type A, Jingke 68-1 strain, ECHO 11, and herpes simplex virus. A stronger inhibitory action was exhibited by a 2% decoction against adenovirus type III, poliomyelitis virus type II, Coxsachie virus group A and B, ECHO 11 group, encephalitis B virus, Jingweiyan I, and herpes simplex I strain; the MIC (minimal inhibitory concentration) against these viruses were 1:1600, 1:400, 1:400, 1:2560, 1:10.240, 1:3200, and 1:51,200, respectively. A 20% solution had a significant inhibitory action against the hepatitis B antigen (HBAg). Active principles I and II of the herb were able to decrease the HBAg titer eightfold. Clinically, it has been used for viral hepatitis, acute inflammatory diseases, neonatal jaundice, and leukopenia.

Isatidis Radix is commonly used in TCM for viral infections. A 50% injection preparation of the herb showed in chicken-embryo and in vitro experiments to have a marked inhibitory action against the influenza virus strains PR8 and Jingke 68-1. In monolayer primary tissue culture of human embryonic renal cells, a 100% decoction of the herb delayed cellular changes caused by Jingke 68-1 and adnovirus type 7. Clinically, it has been used for viral hepatitis, encephalitis B, chickenpox, mumps, viral skin diseases, and influenza.

Rhei Rhizoma's many therapeutic effects have been extensively studied, though here only its anti-viral effects are listed. Strong inhibitory action was exhibited by a decoction of the herb against the influenza virus. The minimum effective dose in chicken embryos was 5mg per embryo. Clinically, it has been used for indigestion, constipation, acute inflammatory diseases, infectious and parasitic diseases, hemorrhaging, and thrombocytopenia (low platelets).

C. Clinical Use

HC Virostatic Formula lowers the HCV load.

D. Package

Each capsule contains 500mg of the formula extracts. One bottle contains 180 capsules, enough for 1 month.

E. Dose

Take 2 capsules, 3 times a day, 10 to 20 minutes before meals.

Circulation Tablet No. 1

Circulation Tablet No. 1 improves blood circulation, especially microcirculation and blood rheology, thereby ensuring that improved or normalized liver function will be sustained. It promotes liver cell regeneration, suppresses fibrosis, and improves overall health.

A. Herbal Composition

Carthami Flos, Persicae Semen, Angelicae Radix, Cnidii Rhizoma, Rehmanniae Radix, Paeoniae rubra Radix, Achyranthis Radix, Citri aurantii Fructus, Bupleuri Radix, Glycyrrhizae Radix, and *Platycodi Radix*

B. Traditional Application

Circulation Tablet No. 1 is modified from the traditional TCM formulas Persica & Achyranthes Combination and Persica & Cnidium Combination. Traditionally, these formulas were used for blood stagnancy (also called blood stasis), with the typical symptoms of dark or purplish tongue, cold hands and feet, dark rings around the eyes, liver palm, spider moles, dry and itchy skin, rashes, lumps, pain, and upper abdominal discomfort.

C. Pharmacology

1. Circulation Tablet No. 1 improves microcirculation: This formula can noticeably ameliorate acute microcirculation disorder induced by macromolecular dextran in rats. It dilates micro-capillaries, accelerates blood flow, and opens more micro-capillary networks. As a result, it increases blood infusion to the tissues and halts the pathology caused by microcirculation disorder. It can promote phagocytosis of macrophages (Kupffer cells) in the liver. It can clear clotting factors in DIC (diffused intravenous clotting) and stop the progress of DIC.

2. Circulation Tablet No. 1 does not prolong PTT or prothrombo time, though it can suppress the clustering of platelets and improve various blood rheological parameters.

3. Circulation Tablet No. 1 improves phagocytosis of macrophages. It can also regulate cellular and humeral immunity.

4. Circulation Tablet No. 1 can noticeably suppress granuloma (fibrosis activities) formation.

D. Clinical Use

Circulation Tablet No. 1 treats chronic hepatitis when used in conjunction with other liver-protecting herbs. It can promote normalization of liver function, shrink enlarged liver and spleen, promote absorption of ascites, and improve overall blood circulation.

Circulation Tablet No. 1 also treats cirrhosis of the liver. The Tianjing Institute of Emergent Medicine in Tianjing, China, used it to treat 18 cases of ascites caused by cirrhosis and found it was very effective.

Besides application in liver diseases, Circulation Tablet No. 1 has been extensively used in internal medicine, gynecology, and surgery for at least 35 clinical conditions.

E. Package

Each tablet contains 500mg of the formula extracts. One bottle contains 180 tablets, enough for 15 days.

F. Dose

Take 4 tablets, 3 times a day with meals.

Circulation Tablet No. 4

Circulation Tablet No. 4 is similar to Circulation Tablet No. 1, though it is used for a maintenance protocol. The major ingredients of Circulation Tablet No. 4 are the same as those of Circulation Tablet No. 1, only the proportions are different.

HerbSom Capsule

HerbSom Capsule is made from the extracts of a centuries-old herbal formula traditionally used for improving sleep.

A. Herbal Composition

Corydalis yanhusao Rhizoma, Zizyphus spinosi Semen, and *Schizandrae Fructus*

B. Clinical Pharmacology

The formula has been studied in teaching hospitals in China. Randomized, insomnia-drug-controlled clinical trials have shown that this formula has definite sleep-inducing effects and improves the quality of sleep as well. In a 374-patient study, improvement in sleep was found to be statistically equivalent to that of methaqualone, an insomnia drug, with far fewer adverse reactions. It is not habit-forming and has no residual effect. The pharmacological data of the herbs contained in this formula show many beneficial effects on the body's cardiovascular and neurological systems. These herbs have no harmful effects on the liver and, in fact, are used in TCM for liver diseases.

C. Package

Each capsule contains 300mg of the extracts of HerbSom Formula, 60 capsules per bottle, enough for 1 month.

D. Dose

Take 2 capsules at bedtime.

Caution: Keep out of reach of children. Don't take while driving a car or operating heavy machinery.

Red Peony Combination

Portal vein hypertension is the central cause of many complications in the advanced stages of liver disease. It can cause ascites, enlargement of the spleen, verices, hemorrhoids, and edema. Reducing portal vein pressure is an important treatment component for advanced hepatitis C.

A. Herbal Composition

Paeoniae rubra Radix, Puerariae Radix, Salviae miltiorrhizae Radix, Persicae Semen, Artemisiae capillaris Herba, and *Aristolochiae fangchi Radix*

B. Clinical Pharmacology

A research hospital in China found that a high dose of extract of *Paeoniae rubra Radix* (red peony root) can significantly reduce portal vein pressure. This herbal extract is the major ingredient of Red Peony Combination.

Aristolochiae fangchi Radix's main active ingredient, hanfangchin A, has been used clinically for cirrhosis caused by viral hepatitis. It can noticeably lower portal vein pressure: 50mg, 3 times a day, taken orally, can dramatically reduce pressure in the portal vein, spleen vein, and superior mesenteric vein. After 1 month of taking this remedy, blood pressure in esophageal varices reduced 11.2 cm H_2O (32%), while in a control group using inderal, the reduction was only 3.3 cm H_2O (9%). The difference was statistically significant. Animal studies found that in a young pig portal vein hypertension model, hanfangchin A can quickly reduce blood pressure in the portal vein. It is an important therapeutic agent for portal vein hypertension in cirrhosis cases. It has been used for treating silicosis and can reverse lung fibrosis. In an animal lung silicosis model using this agent, the treated group showed less collagen in the lungs, the number of silicosis nodules were much fewer, and the fibers were less dense, compared with the control group.

C. Package

Each capsule contains 500mg extracts of the formula. One bottle contains 120 capsules.

D. Dose

Take 4 capsules, 3 times a day or 2g of the granulated formula, 3 times a day, with water, 10 to 20 minutes before meals.

Bitter Melon Capsule

The liver is an important organ in regulating blood sugar. During chronic hepatitis, many patients develop diabetes and hypoglycemia. Bitter Melon Capsule has been successfully used to regulate blood sugar.

A. Herbal Composition

Momordica charantia (bitter melon) and *Fagophyrum tatarium* (bitter buckwheat)

B. Clinical Pharmacology

The two constituent herbs contain active ingredients that can help lower and stabilize blood sugar level. Both have been used for diabetes in Asia and Central and South America for centuries. In China and Southeastern Asia, bitter melon is a commonly consumed vegetable, a testament to its safety as an herbal remedy.

Recently a capsule containing bitter melon and bitter buckwheat has been used in the U.S. and the clinical outcome of its blood-sugar-normalizing effect has proven reliable. It takes about 2 weeks to lower or normalize blood sugar level using Bitter Melon Capsule. Continued use maintains the normalized level.

A 1981 clinical trial in England found that extract of bitter melon fruit significantly improved glucose tolerance in Type II (adult-onset) diabetics. Further testing using a water-soluble extract of bitter melon found that the extract "significantly reduced blood glucose concentrations during oral glucose tolerance tests." Animal studies with normal and diabetic rats and rabbits have shown bitter melon possesses a hypoglycemic (lowering of blood sugar levels) effect. Extract of bitter melon can also stimulate the pancreas to secrete insulin, so it can help Type II diabetics produce more insulin.

Insulin-like molecules in bitter melon extract have physiological effects similar to those of insulin, indicating that it has beneficial effects for Type I (juvenile-onset) diabetics, who do not secrete insulin. Some of the active ingredients of bitter melon can prolong the effects of insulin. Thus the blood-sugar-regulating effects of the herb are gradual and steady, exactly what is necessary to prevent blood sugar swings from low to high and back again. Comparative studies conducted in China found that bitter melon's blood sugar reduction effects were similar to and stronger than those of tolbutamide (D860), a pharmaceutical used to stabilize blood sugar in Type II diabetics.

Bitter buckwheat is used as an absorption medium for bitter melon extract. Bitter buckwheat has also shown hypoglycemic, blood-lipid-reduction, and anti-oxidant effects. When used concurrently, bitter melon and bitter buckwheat show a synergistic relationship.

C. Package

Each capsule contains 500mg of the extracts of bitter melon and bitter buckwheat. Each bottle contains 100 capsules.

D. Dose

Take 3 capsules, 3 times a day, 10 to 20 minutes before meals.

Caution: Pregnant women should not use Bitter Melon Capsule.

AI Capsule No. 3

A. Herbal Composition

Mucunae Caulis, Sargentodoxae Caulis, and *Paederiae Caulis*

B. Clinical Pharmacology

Mucunae Caulis is also known by the botanical name *Spatholobus suberectus Dunn*. In TCM it is said to be bittersweet and warm-propertied. It is used for promoting blood circulation, activating collateral flow, and treating irregular menstruation and lassitude in the loin and legs.

Pharmacological studies found that it can noticeably suppress arthritis caused by formaldehyde in rats. It has sedative and sleep-inducing effects. Clinically, it has been used for amenorrhea and leukemia caused by radiation.

Sargentodoxae Caulis is also known by the botanical name *Sargentodoxa cuncata* (Oliv.) Rehd et Wils. In TCM it is considered bitter and mild, with antiphlogistic (detoxification) and detumescemce (subsidence of swelling) effects. Moreover, the herb promotes blood circulation and activates collateral flow. Clinically, it is used for treating acute and chronic appendicitis, irregular menstruation, and rheumatism. Pharmacological studies found it can suppress various bacteria, such as *Staphylococcus aureus*, *Streptococcus*, and *Pseudomonas aeruginosa*. In modern clinical applications, it has been used to treat leprosy, rheumatic arthritis, and appendicitis.

Paederiae Caulis is also known by the botanical name *Paederia scandens* (Lour.) Merr. TCM considers it to be mild-propertied and sweet with a slightly bitter aftertaste. It possesses antirheumatic, digestant, antitussive, mucolytic, and analgesic properties. It is used to treat rheumatic pains, injuries due to impact, fractures, contusions and strains, eczema, pyogenic infections, and ulcers of the skin.

Pharmacological studies found that it has analgesic and sedative actions. It can elevate the pain threshold and inhibit spontaneous activity in mice and prolong pentobarbital sodium-induced sleep. The total alkaloids of this herb inhibited the contraction of isolated intestine and antagonized spasm due to acetylcholine and histamine. The herb possesses expectorant, antibacterial, hypotensive, corticoid-cortisone-like, and local anesthetic actions. It has a high LD_{50} and has virtually no toxicity. Clinically, it has been used for skin diseases (eczema, neurodermatitis, and lepromatous leprosy) and respiratory tract diseases (bronchitis and whooping cough).

C. Package

Each capsule contains 100mg of extracts of the formula. One bottle contains 50 capsules.

D. Dose

Take 1 or 2 capsules, 3 times a day; or follow healthcare provider's advice.

Capillaris Combination

This is a very old and famous formula formulated by the Chinese medical sage Zhang Zhongjing about 1,800 years ago. It was first described in his book *Shang Han Lun* (Treatise on Febrile Diseases). This time-honored formula has a wide range of applications.

A. Herbal Composition

Artemisiae capillaris Herba, Gardeniae Fructus, and *Rhei Rhizoma*.

B. Clinical Pharmacology

Regarding the formula's traditional use in TCM, Capillaris Combination clears "dampness-heat" type jaundice, manifesting as bright yellow eyes and skin; oliguria with dark yellow color; greasy, yellow tongue coating; and smooth, rapid pulse.

Artemisiae capillaris Herba has been discussed in Gall Formula No. 1. *Rhei Rhizoma*'s pharmacological actions are discussed above in Virostatic Formula.

The pharmacological effects of Capillaris Combination have been well-studied, and it has been found to possess cholagogic (increasing flow of bile to the intestine) and choleretic (facilitating bile secretion) effects. Intraduodenal administration of alcohol extracts to rats can increase up to 51% of the bile collected and increase the solid composition of the bile 85%. It can also be used against the cholestatic (arrest of bile excretion) factor's effect in rats. Its choleretic effects are mainly due to increasing the secretion of the bile in the micro-bile ducts. Bile excretion is probably promoted by the relaxation of the Oddi's sphincter following increase of intraductal pressure consequent to increase of bile secreted by liver cells.

Capillaris Combination has liver-protective effects and can reduce liver damage caused by ANIT (alpha-naphthyl isothiocyanate). While using this formula, AKP, T-BILI, ALT, and AST elevations caused by ANIT all improved dramatically. It is especially effective in improving T-BILI. Histological examination revealed that hypertrophy of the micro-bile duct cells, necrosis of liver cells, and inflammatory cell infiltration were much milder in the Capillaris Combination-treated group, as compared with the control group. Liver glycogen and RNA content were normalized or almost recovered, and ALT activity was markedly reduced with Capillaris Combination.

C. Clinical Use

Capillaris Combination is used for acute or chronic viral hepatitis, jaundice, and gallbladder inflammation.

D. Package

Capillaris Combination is available in capsule and granular form. One bottle contains 100 capsules or 100g of the granulated formula.

E. Dose

Take 4 capsules or 2g of the granulated formula, 3 times a day, with water, 10 to 20 minutes before meals.

Ginseng & Atractylodes Formula

Ginseng & Atractylodes Formula was created by the National Medical Bureau of the Song Dynasty, about 1,000 years ago.

A. Herbal Composition

Ginseng Radix, Dioscoreae Rhizoma, Dolichoris album Semen, Coicis Semen, Nelumbinis Semen, Atractylodis macro-

cephalae Rhizoma, Poriae Alba, Glycyrrhizae Radix, Amomi Fructus, and *Platycodi Radix.*

B. Clinical Pharmacology

Traditionally, Ginseng & Atractylodes Formula was used for strengthening digestion and qi (vital energy). It is used for diarrhea; poor appetite; emaciation; and white, greasy tongue coating.

Pharmacological studies have found that Ginseng & Atractylodes Formula can improve absorption in the intestinal track. Administration of a decoction of the formula can increase water and chloride absorption in the intestines of rabbits under anesthesia. In vitro tests found that high doses of the formula suppress intestinal movement and small doses increase the movement. It is an antagonist to the spastic effects of acetylcholine on the intestine.

Ginseng & Atractylodes Formula treats chronic gastritis, ulcerative enterophthisis, chronic pancreatitis with diarrhea, chronic nephritis with persistence of proteinuria, and hepatitis.

C. Package

Ginseng & Atractylodes is available in capsule and granular form. One bottle contains 100 capsules or 100g of the granulated formula.

D. Dose

Take 4 capsules or 2g of the granulated formula, 3 times a day, with water, 10 to 20 minutes before meals.

Stephania & Astragalus Combination

Stephania & Astragalus Combination was formulated by the Chinese medical sage Zhang Zhongjing about 1,800 years ago. This time-honored formula was first described in his book *Jin Gau Yao Lue* (Synopsis of Prescriptions from the Golden Chamber).

A. Herbal Composition

Aristolochiae fangchi Radix, Astragali Radix, Atractylodis macrocephalae Rhizoma, Glycyrrhizae Radix, Zizyphi jujubae Fructus, and *Zingiberis Rhizoma*

B. Clinical Pharmacology

Aristolochiae fangchi Radix, the main ingredient of this formula, has been discussed in the section on Red Peony Combination.

Stephania & Astragalus Combination has diuretic effects and is used mainly to treat water retention, though also for rheumatism, joint pain, feeling of bodily heaviness, excessive sweating, nephritis, and idiopathic edema.

C. Package

Stephania & Astragalus Combination is available in capsule and granular form. One bottle contains 100 capsules or 100g of granulated formula.

D. Dose

Take 4 capsules or 2g of the granulated formula, 3 times a day, with water, 10 to 20 minutes before meals.

Yunnan Paiyao Capsule

This well-known folk medicine has been widely used in China and Southeastern Asia with excellent therapeutic results, especially for hemostatic (stopping bleeding) treatment.

A. Herbal Composition

Proprietary information

B. Clinical Pharmacology

1. Hemostatic effects: Yunnan Paiyao Capsule has obvious hemostatic effects, as it can quickly halt bleeding in animal models. In rat liver injury model, rabbit liver injury model, and rabbit large artery injury model, bleeding stopped almost immediately after this formula was administered. It can dramatically reduce clotting time in humans and rabbits. Hemostatic effects generally begin a half hour after administration and peak 2 to 3 hours after administration. These effects can last for more than 4 hours. The hemostatic effect is due to the permeability change of platelet cell membranes, which prompts release of clotting factors.

2. Anti-inflammatory effects: Yunnan Paiyao Capsule can suppress inflammation in animal models. The strength of its anti-inflammatory effect is similar to or stronger than that of cortico-steroids.

3. Analgesic and anti-neoplastic effects.

C. Clinical Use

Yunnan Paiyao Capsule is mainly used for gastrointestinal bleeding, gastritis, ulcerative colitis, and lung and stomach cancers.

D. Package

Each capsule contains 500mg of the herbal extract, with 16 capsules per plate.

E. Dose

Take 1 capsule, 4 times a day, 10 to 20 minutes before meals and before bed.

HerbZac Capsule

A. Herbal Composition

Hypericum (St. John's wort), *Acori Rhizoma* (acorus), *Camellia Sinensis* (green tea), *Menthae Herba* (mentha arvensis), and *Schisandra fructus.*

B. Clinical Pharmacology

Hypericin is the active ingredeint of St. John's wort. This herb has been used for centuries to treat mental disorders and is very popular in Europe. In Germany it is the most popular treatment for depression. In China, *Hypericum* has been used for treating viral hepatitis. It has liver-protective effects and can help lower liver enzyme levels.

Camellia sinensis (green tea) contains derivatives of xanthin, such as theophyline and caffeine, that carry the main pharmacological effects of green tea. They have excitatory effects on the higher central nervous system and have mental incitation effects to make people think faster. They can alleviate fatigue. They are also antioxidants, which protect the cell membrane from viral infection.

Acorus has both sedative and incitative effects. Its effects are determined by the state of the central nervous system of the patient. When it is depressed, the herb can be an incitantia and when it is excited, the herb has sedative effects.

Menthae Herba in TCM is used for "promoting circulation of qi and alleviation of mental depression."

C. Clinical Use

For depression and anxiety.

D. Package

Each capsule contains 500mg of the extract of the formula and each bottle contains 90 capsules.

E. Dose

Take 3 capsules twice a day, morning and noon. Do not take in the evening.

SINGLE HERBS

Glycyrrihzin Capsule

Glycyrrhizin (GL) is an important herbal remedy for treating viral hepatitis, since it acts on several pathological aspects of the disease.

A. Original Herb

Glycyrrhizae uralensis Fisch (licorice root)

B. Chemical Composition

GL consists of triterpenes glycyrrhizin and glycyrrhetinic acid, usually as salts of glycyrrhizic acid and ammonia, calcium, potassium, iron, or barium. The glycyrrhizin capsule we use is a potassium salt of glycyrrhizic acid.

C. Traditional Use

Licorice is the most frequently used herb in traditional Chinese medicine (TCM) and has been extensively studied. TCM classifies licorice as a sweet, mild herb and uses it to supplement the body, clear "latent heat," regulate stomach functions, expectorate the lungs, and invigorate the spleen. It has been used as an antipyretic, detoxicant, and anti-inflammatory. Many TCM formulas use licorice as a corrective adjutant and harmonizing ingredient. Clinically, it is used for cough, palpitation, stomachache, peptic ulcer, phyogenic infection, and skin rashes.

D. Pharmacology

GL has the following pharmacological actions that can be used in treating hepatitis C.

1. Anti-viral effects: GL induces the generation of interferon-gamma in test animals and in humans. It can prolong the survival of mice following injection with hepatitis virus MHV. In rabbits, it can inhibit virus proliferation.

   Seventeen hospitals in China have studied the therapeutic effects of GL on 300 cases of hepatitis B. The clinical curative rate was 44% and the effectiveness rate was 77%, with 41% of the patients seeing their HBeAg serum positive status convert to negative. Treating viral hepatitis with GL can significantly shorten the disease course, accelerate recovery of liver function, normalize ALT and AST, and turn HBeAg to negative in about 40% of patients. Studies in Japan have confirmed these effects.

2. Protecting and healing liver cells from chemical and biological injuries: GL can alleviate histological disorder due to inflammation and restore liver structure and function from damage due to carbon tetrachloride. The effects include lowering ALT (SGPT): 64% with normalized ALT following administration in a Japanese study and 87% in a study conducted in China. GL can reduce degeneration and necrosis, and recover glycogen and RNA of liver cells. Experimental hepatitis and cirrhosis studies on rats found that GL can promote the regeneration of liver cells and inhibit fibrosis. It can also reduce gamma-globulin and interstitial inflammation in the liver.

3. Other pharmacological effects: Anti-allergic, anti-inflammatory, and detoxifying activities are all important for its use in treating viral hepatitis. Its anti-allergic and anti-inflammatory activities resemble the activities of glucocorticoid, since GL maintains the level of active corticoid in the blood and increases endogenous corticoid by inhibiting deactivation of glucocorticoid in the liver. Further, GL promotes the regeneration of inflammatory tissue in contrast with glucocorticoid, which inhibits regeneration. GL also inhibits the release of histamine from mast cells.

E. Package

Each capsule contains 150mg of GL and other herbal extracts, and each bottle contains 60 capsules.

F. Dose

Take 1 capsule, 2 times a day, 10 to 20 minutes before breakfast and dinner.

Caution: Although licorice is a non-toxic herb, long-term use can cause some adverse reactions in about 20% of patients. Edema, elevated blood pressure, low blood potassium, dizziness, and fatigued limbs may be seen. Patients with hypertension (high blood pressure) should not take Glycyrrhizin Capsule.

Ligustrin Capsule

A. Original Herb

Ligustrum Fructus (*Ligustrum lucidum Ait*)

B. Traditional Use

Traditional Chinese medicine uses ligustrum as a tonic for the liver and kidneys, principally as a treatment of symptoms associated with "yin deficiencies," such as dizziness, blurred vision, tinnitus, premature graying of hair, and low-back ache.

C. Chemical Composition

Ligustrin is a highly purified extract of *Ligustrum lucidum Fructus*. Its major chemical component is oleanolic acid. Other components include acetyloleanolic acid, betulin, lupeol, salidroside, mannitol, oleic acid, linolenic acid, and palmitic acid.

D. Pharmacological Actions

Ligustrin protects the liver from chemical and biological injuries through the following actions.

1. Ligustrin helps lower the liver enzyme ALT (SGPT) level. In experimental cirrhosis studies, ligustrin inhibited degeneration and reduced necrosis of liver

cells. It can increase glycogen in the liver, accelerate repair of necrosed tissue, and promote regeneration of liver cells. It can also inhibit inflammation and collagen formation.

2. Ligustrin raises the WBC count and is used to treat leukopenia caused by radiation and chemotherapy.

3. In clinical trials for treating acute or chronic hepatitis, it can rapidly reduce ALT, AST, and jaundice; it has a 90% clinical cure rate for acute icterohepatitis and a 70% effectiveness rate for chronic hepatitis.

4. Ligustrin has immune-regulatory effects, specifically, it promotes lymphoblast cell transformation, suppresses Ts cells, increases Th cells, and promotes phagocytosis of macrophages.

5. Ligustrin can increase coronary blood flow.

6. Acute and chronic toxicity tests have shown that ligustrin has very low toxicity. After injecting dogs with 50mg/kg IV and mice with 5mg/20g IV, 24 hours of observation found no adverse reactions. After injecting rabbits with 50mg/kg IP daily for 6 to 12 weeks, no heart, liver, or kidney disorders were found.

E. Clinical Applications

Ligustrin is applied in the clinic to treat acute and chronic hepatitis, leukopenia caused by radiation or chemotherapy, and chronic fatigue syndrome.

F. Package

Each capsule contains 300mg of ligustrin extract. Each bottle contains 90 capsules, enough for 1 month.

G. Dose

Take 1 capsule, 3 times a day, 10 to 20 minutes before meals.

Olive Leaf

A. Original Plant

The leaf of *Canarium album* (Lour.) *Raeusch*

B. Chemical Composition of Active Ingredients

Oleuopein is the extract of the olive leaf, and its active ingredient is elenolic acid.

C. Pharmacology

TCM considers olive leaf bitter, astringent, sour, and mild-propertied. It is used for clearing the lungs and detoxifying.

Pharmacological studies found that it has powerful anti-bacterial effects. Elenolic acid has a very wide anti-viral spectrum. It was found to suppress herpes, influenza, and the common cold. Olive leaf decoction has been used against HIV infections.

D. Preparations

Olive leaf decoction: Packed in a 1-pound bag for a 1-month supply. To make a decoction, soak half of the bag (0.5 lb.) in a gallon of water and slowly cook in a crock pot at 175 to 185° F for about 12 hours. Filter out the olive leaves and store the liquid in the refrigerator. Drink 3 ounces, twice a day between meals.

Olivessence Capsule

A. Original herb

Canarium album (Lour.) Raeusch and the leaf of this plant is used.

B. Chemical Composition of Active Ingredients

Oleuopein is the extract of the olive leaf, which is a phenolic compound. Its active ingredient is elenolic acid. The extract used in this capsule contains 18% oleuopein, which is for professional use and is the highest concentration available.

C. Pharmacology

In TCM, it is considered to have a bitter, sour taste and mild property. It is used for clearing the lungs and detoxification.

Pharmacological studies found that it has powerful anti-bacterial, anti-viral, and antiprotozoal effects. In vitro experiments with calcium elenolate, a salt of elenolic acid, demonstrated an effect against viruses, bacteria, and protozoans. When tested with viral cultures, it suppressed the following viruses: herpes, vaccinia, pseudorabies, Newcastle, Coxsacloe A21, polio 1, 2, and 3, vesicular stomititus, Moloney Murine leukemia, influenza, and common cold.

Animal experiments showed that the compound was tolerated very well, with no serious adverse reactions. Clinically, this herbal remedy has been used for HIV infections.

F. Package

Each capsule contains 500mg of olive leaf extract. Each bottle contains 60 capsules, for a 1-month supply.

G. Dose

Take 1 capsule twice a day.

Cordyceps Capsule

A. Original Herb and Traditional Use

Cordyceps sinensis is the stroma of *Cordyceps sinensis* (Berk.) Sacc. (Ascomycetes) together with the host larva of *Hepialus armoricanus Oberthur* (Hepialidae). Originally, it was found only in a small area of Qinghai province of China. Since it is very rare and expensive, Chinese scientists have found a way to cultivate it and make it more accessible through more than 20 years of intensive study. The cultivated version of this product is made from the dried mycelia powder of *Cephalosporium sinensis* Chen. sp., now isolated from fresh *Cordyceps sinensis* (Berk) Sacc through submerged fermentation in a liquid medium. It is available in a homogenous, high-quality, and consistently effective form. Its capsule version is easy to administer.

According to TCM, cordyceps is considered warm-propertied with a sweet, acrid taste. It nourishes the lungs; tonifies the kidneys, vital essence, and vital energy (qi); balances the body; and resolves phlegm. It is used to treat general debility following prolonged illness, especially in elderly patients.

B. Chemical Composition

Among other constituents, cordyceps contains 17 amino acids, 10 trace elements, D-mannitol, and ergosterol.

C. Pharmacology

The Beijing Institute of Materia Medica of the Chinese Medical Academy made extensive pharmacological studies of *Cordyceps sinensis* and found that the cultivated version has the same chemical components and the same physiological effects as the natural product. Its remarkable therapeutic effects have been confirmed in many controlled, well-designed studies carried out by medical schools in Beijing, Shanghai, Nanjing, and other provinces of China. Its therapeutic effects on the liver have been extensively studied in China. Its toxicity is very low; in therapeutic doses, virtually no toxicity has been observed. Besides its therapeutic effects on the liver, cordyceps has the following pharmacological actions: immune-system-enhancement, anti-inflammatory, anti-asthmatic, elevation of high-density lipoproteins (HDL), reduction of blood cholesterol, reduction of platelet aggregation, stimulation of blood supply to the heart and brain, anti-neoplastic (anti-tumor), and enhancement of phagocytosis of macrophages.

D. Clinical Applications

1. Regarding the treatment of chronic viral hepatitis, the effectiveness rate of *Cordyceps sinensis* was reportedly more than 80% in a 256-case clinical study. Cordyceps can lower ALT, improve liver function, relieve symptoms, and increase albumin. Cordyceps has also been used for cirrhosis caused by viral hepatitis. In 22 cases, following 3 months of use, 17 patients saw their albumin levels increase. Among 17 patients with ascites, 12 saw their ascites disappear, while 5 cases reduced their ascites. Cordyceps can reduce enlarged spleen and reduce

pressure in the portal vein. It can also dramatically improve stamina.

2. Immune deficiency caused by viral infection, chemotherapy, radiation therapy, or complications following surgery or major illness are effectively treated with *Cordyceps sinensis.*

3. Chronic respiratory track infections, asthma, bronchitis, and tuberculosis can be effectively treated with cordyceps, which can also be used to prevent flu and the common cold.

4. Impotence, premature ejaculation, low libido, low sperm count and activity, irregular menstruation, and leukorrhea are all effectively treated with *Cordyceps sinensis.*

5. Constitutional asthenia (weakness) associated with cancer, AIDS, TB, convalescence, and wasting syndrome are all benefited with the use of cordyceps.

6. High blood lipoproteins and hypertension can be treated with cordyceps.

7. Cordyceps treats arrhythmia, especially slow-type arrhythmia. It can accelerate atrioventricular conduction, enhance or regulate sinus rhythm, inhibit ectopic rhythm, and improve heart function.

E. Package

Each capsule contains 300mg of *Cordyceps sinensis* mycelia. One bottle contains 90 capsules.

F. Dose

Take 2 capsules, 3 times a day, 10 to 20 minutes before meals.

Allicin Capsule

A. Original Herb

Allii sativum Bulbus (garlic)

B. Chemical Composition

Allicin is the highly purified and concentrated essence of garlic, allitridi.

C. Pharmacology

Pharmacological studies have found that allicin has a very wide spectrum of anti-infectious properties. It is effective against bacteria, mycobacteria, fungi, protozoa, and certain viruses. It is potent enough to treat many common infections and has been used for more than 20 years in China to treat bacillary dysentery, amebic dysentery, deep fungal infections, whooping cough, endobronchial tuberculosis, oxyuriasis, and trichomonas vaginitis. For most of these conditions, the cure rate is more than 80%. Recent studies conducted by the AIDS Research Alliance in Los Angeles found that allicin can be used to treat cryptosporidiosis, a diarrheal disease caused by protozoa of the genus *Cryptosporidium* and commonly seen in AIDS patients. We have been using this substance successfully to treat many infectious diseases in our practice. It also benefits the cardiovascular system and is a strong anti-oxidant.

Allicin is a very safe herbal remedy. Its only drawback, at least to some, is its odor. The LD_{50} of allicin is 134.9 times its therapeutic dose. In animal studies, long-term usage of allicin has not produced any pathological changes.

D. Package

Each capsule contains 20mg of allicin. One bottle contains 30 capsules. The capsules used in our clinic are of the highest potency available on the market. Until just recently, the highest potency available was only 2.5 to 3mg per capsule. Allicin Capsule is in time-release form and is enterically coated, which helps to keep the blood level of allicin stable and to reduce stimulation to the stomach.

E. Dose

For prevention, 1 capsule per day. To treat infections, 2 or 3 capsules, 3 times a day, with or before meals.

Allicin Solution

A. Original Herb

Allii sativum Bulbus (garlic)

B. Chemical Composition

Allicin is the highly purified and concentrated essence of garlic, allitridi.

C. Pharmacology

Same as Allicin Capsule (see previous formula)

D. Package

Each vial contains 30mg of allicin in 2ml of liquid. One box contains 10 vials.

E. Dose

Take 1 to 2 vials a day, diluted with at least 8 ounces of water (1 cup) per vial, with or before meals.

Coptin Tablet

Coptin is an herbal remedy with various anti-infectious properties.

A. Original Herb

Coptis chinensis Franch

B. Chemical Composition

The major chemical ingredient of *Coptis chinensis* is umbellatine.

C. Pharmacology

Pharmacological studies found that coptin has various anti-infectious properties.

1. Anti-bacterial actions: coptin can strongly suppress *Staphylococcus aureus, Streptococcus, Pneumococcus, Vibrio comma, Anthrax bacillus,* and *Bacillus dysenteriae*. It can also suppress *Hay bacillus, Pneumobacillus, Bacillus diphtheriae, Bordetella pertussis, Brucellaceae,* and *Mycobacterium tuberculosis*. Its potency is roughly equal to or stronger than that of sulfanilamide and slightly weaker than that of streptomycin and chloramphenicol.

2. Anti-viral actions: coptin can suppress influenza viruses and Newcastle disease virus in vitro.

3. Other anti-pathogen actions: coptin can suppress *Ameba, Chlamydi trachomatis, Trichomonad,* and *Leptospira*.

4. Besides anti-infectious effects, coptin has anti-cancer, anti-radiation, and blood-sugar-regulatory effects. In treating chronic hepatitis, its cholagogic (bile-secretion-facilitating) effect is especially useful.

5. Toxicity: coptin is a very safe herbal remedy, with virtually no side effects. Long-term use has not caused any adverse reactions or accumulative toxicity. LD_{50} for rats is 205mg/kg.

D. Clinical Use

1. Coptin is a wide-spectrum anti-infectious agent and has been used for treating bacterial infections such as abscess, bacillary dysentery, and gastritis.

2. Coptin can relieve symptoms of chronic gallbladder inflammation and reduce bilirubin levels, with an effectiveness rate of around 88.2%.

3. Respiratory infections, such as bronchitis, sinusitis, and tonsillitis, can be effectively treated with coptin.

4. Protozoa infections, such as amebic dysentery and trichomonas vaginitis, as well as yeast infection (specifically, candidiasis), can be treated with coptin.

5. Coptin has also been used to treat Type II diabetes, cardiac arrhythmia, and hypertension.

E. Package

One tablet contains 100mg of coptin. One bottle contains 50 tablets.

F. Dose

Take 2 or 3 tablets, 3 times a day, 10 to 20 minutes before meals.

Rhubarbin Tablet

A. Original Herb

Rhei Rhizoma (rhubarb root)

B. Chemical Composition

Extracts made by alcohol extraction of this herb contain aloe-emodin, rhein, and chrysophanol.

C. Pharmacology

Pharmacological studies have found that rhubarb root extracts have various anti-infectious effects. Rhubarb can effectively suppress *Staphylococcus, Anthrax bacillus, Bacillus dysenteriae, Streptococcus,* and *E. coli.* It is especially effective for *Staphylococcus* and *Streptococcus.* It also has anti-cancer and immune-regulatory effects. Its strong purgative and laxative effects can be used to treat constipation.

Among rhubarb's 3 major constituents, rhein has the strongest anti-infection and antibacterial effects. Chrysophanol has homeostatic (stopping bleeding) effects and is often used for bleeding in the gastrointestinal system.

Rhubarb's toxicity is very low: its LD_{50} is 250 to 500mg/kg, while chrysophanol's LD_{50} is 10g/kg, making it very safe.

D. Clinical Applications

Rhubarbin Tablet has been used for more than 48 clinical conditions, including acute and chronic gallbladder inflammation, pancreas inflammation, gastritis, and constipation.

E. Package

Each tablet contains 500mg of rhubarb root extract. One bottle contains 50 tablets.

F. Dose

Take 2 tablets, 3 times a day, 10 to 20 minutes before meals, or follow the advice of your practitioner.

5

Frequently Asked Questions

Hepatitis C virus was identified just a decade ago, so hepatitis C is a newly defined disease. I am introducing a foreign medical system to treat it. Naturally, there will be many questions about my approach. Since Dr. Andrew Weil recommended my protocol in his newsletter *Self Healing*, I have received many letters concerning the treatment of HCV and HBV with Chinese medicinal herbs. Here are some of the most commonly asked questions.

Q: I plan to have a blood panel done prior to beginning herbal treatment and again after two to three months. Would you like to see the test results?

A: It is a very good idea to have a baseline test result to use for comparison with subsequent results. I strongly recommend every patient have a baseline test before beginning herbal treatment. Two to three months of taking herbs is usually enough time to improve or normalize liver function for most people. Tests should then be repeated every two to three months to monitor the progress of the herbal treatment. I like to collect clinical data on our patients (chemical panel tests including liver function profile and viral load), so that I can better evaluate their conditions and recommend the next step in the treatment process.

Q: I have consulted with my doctor, and he is willing to work with me to monitor my liver function during herbal treatment. Is this okay with you?

A: Of course. It is very good to have a conventional medical doctor monitor your progress during herbal treatment. We encourage everyone in our program to remain under the care of a conventional medical doctor. Please inform your primary physician of your herbal treatment. If your doctor has any questions, he or she is welcome to call me.

Q: Can you explain a little about the composition of Chinese herbal formulas?

A: Most Chinese herbal formulas are made from a combination of 8 to 12 herbs that are categorized as emperor herb(s), minister herb(s), assistant herb(s), and servant herb(s). Emperor and minister herbs are synergistic and perform major pharmacological actions. Assistant herbs mitigate the possible side effects of the emperor and minister herbs, while servant herbs direct the actions of the other herbs to target organs. The recommended herbal formulas used in our clinic adhere to these principles and are therefore well balanced.

Single-herb formulas, such as Ligustrin Capsule and Glycyrrhizin Capsule, are formulated according to pharmacological properties of the herb and its active ingredients.

The recommended herbal formulas are made of herbal extracts, so you don't need to boil them to make a decoction. They are available in tablet, capsule, and/or granular form, which makes taking them convenient and unobjectionable as far as taste and odor are concerned. Every batch of herbal product is standardized to ensure uniform potency and quality. Their effects are predictable and can be replicated.

Q: How long am I to take these herbs?

A: Herb Group I (Hepa Formula No. 2, Ligustrin Capsule, Glycyrrhizin Capsule, and Circulation Tablet No. 1) and Herb Group II (same as Group I, except without Glycyrrhizin Capsule) are designed to normalize liver enzyme levels and heal liver inflammation. Healing inflammation is the most important step in breaking the vicious progression of inflammation, scar formation, and cirrhosis. It is an important step in improving the poor prognosis for chronic hepatitis C. In most patients (about 80%), inflammation can be improved within two to three months. If a patient shows three consecutive normal ALT readings within one year and every reading was taken two to three months apart, we can safely say that liver inflammation is well under control. The patient can then switch to a maintenance protocol to keep ALT normal for at least one to two more years. This will give the liver a chance to regenerate. At the same time, treatment also focuses on lowering the HCV load to reduce virus replication. Once liver functions have normalized, the focus shifts to the prevention of cirrhosis. In short, herbal treatment should last at least one to two years.

Q: Do these herbs eliminate the hepatitis virus?

A: These herbs can suppress the HCV and HBV viruses or block their replication in two ways.

First, the herbs eliminate the virus through regulating immunity. In viral infections, our bodies eliminate viruses mainly through immune reactions. Extracts of Chinese medicinal herbs, such as *Cordyceps sinensis, Sophorae sub-prostratae Radix, Sophorae Radix, Glycyrrhizae Radix,* and *Polyporus umbellatus Pers,* work as immune regulators that restore immune function. And a healthier immune system does a better job of eliminating the virus.

Second, some herbs have been studied for their direct anti-HBV effects (most of the work has been done on hepatitis B virus). In the test tube, *Thlapsi Herba, Rhei Rhizoma, Polygoni cuspidati Rhizoma, Blechni Rhizoma, Houttuyniae Herba,* and *Phellodendri Cortex* can suppress HBsAg, the HBV virus' surface antigen. In clinical treatment, these herbs can convert HBsAg to negative in about 20 to 40% of patients.

In evaluating HBV's infectious activities and replication, HBV DNAP (DNA polymerase) is an important parameter in determining HBV's reproduction rate. The following herbs have been found to suppress HBV DNAP activity by more than 50%: *Chaenomelis Fructus, Salviae miltiorrhizae Radix, Prunellae Spica, Gardeniae Fructus, Moutan radicis Cortex, Paeoniae rubra Radix, Lithospermi Radix, Coptis Rhizoma, Artemisiae ching-hao Herba, Lonicerae Flos, Thlapsi Herba, Polygoni cuspidate Rhizoma, Pulsatillae Radix, Taraxaci Herba, Sophorae sub-prostratae Radix, Scutellariae Radix,* and *Isatidis Radix,* among others. Many of these herbs play key roles in the recommended treatment protocol.

Olive leaf, which is also used in my clinic to treat hepatitis, has been studied extensively for its wide-spectrum anti-viral properties. It has been used for HIV, herpes, and hepatitis.

I cannot promise that every patient will see the total elimination of HCV or HBV virus through the use of these herbs. I have seen, however, that after the recommended herbal treatment, the majority of our patients see their HCV viral load (measured by a quantitative HCV RNA PCR test) decline to a low level (lower than one million/ml) and stabilize there.

Q: Do I automatically receive the next month's order? If not, when should I reorder?

A: Since response to treatment varies from person to person, you will not automatically be sent the next order. Please order your next supply two to three weeks in advance to allow plenty of time for it to reach you. HepaPro Corporation of California is the exclusive distributor. You can contact them at 1-888-788- HEPA (4372).

Q: Can this herbal treatment be harmful or toxic to the liver or any other organs?

A: The herbal products used in the hepatitis C protocols described in this book have been tested for acute and long-term toxicity and have been found to be virtually non-toxic. They have been tested in animal and clinical studies and have shown liver-protective, anti-viral, and anti-inflammatory properties. They show no harmful effects on any organ. Indeed, they have been found to have beneficial effects on the heart, kidneys, brain, and stomach. For their pharmacological features, please read the pharmacological data found in Chapter 4.

One herbal product, Glycyrrhizin Capsule, may cause blood pressure elevation in 20% of people. Should this occur, use of this herb should be discontinued. This effect is reversible; following discontinuation, blood pressure will return to normal.

Q: Can the herbal treatment cause an upset stomach?

A: The herbs used in hepatitis C protocols usually do not cause an upset stomach. Very rarely, though, a person may have an allergic reaction to one of the herbs. The granular form of Hepa Formula No. 3 is quite acidic. If you have chronic stomach illness, e.g. ulcers, you may experience an upset stomach. Other than this, after observing many patients under treatment, we have not noticed any adverse reactions. AI Capsule No. 3 and Circulation Tablet No. 1 should be taken with food to avoid possible stimulation of the mucus membrane of the stomach.

Q: Since taking the herbs, I've been experiencing discomfort—a pinching or burning sensation—in the liver area. Is this normal?

A: In a chronic disease course, when a new treatment is started, some patients will temporarily feel worse than they did prior to treatment. A new treatment causes the old imbalance of the body to become disturbed. This may cause some discomfort. Don't worry, this will soon pass.

Q: I eat only two meals a day. Can the herbs be taken without food for one dose? If not, should I only take them twice?

A: The herbs can be taken without food, though this may cause stomach discomfort in some patients. With or without food, you still need at least a cup of water to dissolve the herbs in your stomach.

If your schedule precludes taking herbs three times a day, you can divide the noon dose in half and add half to your morning and half to your evening doses. Do not reduce your overall daily dose.

Q: What role do height and weight play in prescribing dosage?

A: The herbal dosage does have something to do with weight, but not as strictly as is the case with chemical drugs. If your weight falls into the normal range, a normal dose is prescribed. Only those patients who are extremely over- or underweight need to increase or decrease dosages.

Q: In case I do not belong to the 80% of patients who respond well to herbal treatment, what am I to do?

A: Clinical treatment is a statistical phenomenon; not everybody responds to a treatment in the same way or within the same time frame. Such factors as body constitution, general health, lifestyle, and dedication to the treatment protocol may affect outcome. About 20% of patients will not see improvement after taking either the Group I or Group II herbal protocols. For them, a second line of individualized herbal remedies will be used. Such patients should visit our office to have one-on-one consultations, so that herbs targeted to their individual needs can be prescribed.

Q: Can these herbs help someone who already has cirrhosis?

A: Herbal remedies have been used to treat cirrhosis. I have treated patients with cirrhosis, enlarged or shrunken livers, enlarged spleens, and even ascites (water in the abdomen, which is a sign of a severely compromised state). At this stage, patients usually have a mildly elevated liver enzyme level, yellowish conjunctiva, liver palms, spider moles, and varices. By using herbal protocols to normalize liver function and reduce inflammation, pressure in the portal vein decreases and the spleen shrinks. By improving protein synthesis, albumin level increases, which raises the osmotic pressure of the blood. The water in the abdomen can then be reabsorbed. Patients will also see their liver palms and spider moles disappear. At the same time, herbs to eliminate water through the urine and bowel movement can be used. Cirrhotic animal model studies found that glycyrrhizin and cordyceps can soften the liver and reduce collagen in the cirrhotic liver. I have also used herbal treatments for silicosis (miner's lung, fibrosis of the lungs caused by silicon inhalation) to treat cirrhosis and have found that cirrhosis can be partially reversed, especially in the early stages. For those already awaiting a liver transplant, herbal treatment can improve overall health and can prolong waiting time.

Q: How significant is the viral load test? Why do I sometimes see such dramatic shifts in my viral load readings? Why does my liver enzyme level sometimes show improvement at the same time as the HCV load is getting worse?

A: HCV is a cytopathic and immunopathic virus. It can directly cause liver damage and can also cause immune dysfunction, which in turn can cause liver damage. From pathological studies, we know that most liver damage is due to inadequate immune response. The damage directly caused by HCV replication is minimal. To illustrate this point, note that following liver transplant, due to the use of strong immune suppressive drugs to prevent rejection, viral load becomes very high, even though the new liver is not proportionally damaged. In short, viral load is not closely related to liver damage. Therefore, sometimes you will see your liver enzyme levels improve or normalize, even though your HCV load may still be high.

Moreover, viral load tests are still not very accurate and have not been endorsed by the FDA as a diagnostic procedure. Every lab has its own techniques and calibration methods, making comparisons between labs virtually meaningless. The HCV load of one of my patients tested 156,000 at one lab, and the very next day at another lab the reading was more than 5,000,000. The National Institutes of Health consider quantitative PCR/branched DNA tests to be of unproven value. In order for these tests to have any meaning, they must be done by the same lab, using the same techniques and calibrations. Only then can lab results be used as a reference to evaluate treatment progress.

Viral load can fluctuate and is often affected by mental and physical stress. Any illness, such as the flu, a cold, sinusitis, or sore throat, can elevate the viral load, as can mental and emotional stress. In order to keep your viral load at a low, stable level, pay attention to your overall health.

Q: How significant is a liver biopsy? How often should I have a biopsy performed?

A: A liver biopsy is the most direct way to evaluate liver damage. Even so, according to the Consensus Statement of the National Institutes of Health, the usefulness of serial biopsies in monitoring progression of liver disease is questionable. It is an invasive procedure that can cause morbidity (injury or disease). It is also expensive. This said, patients who have had hepatitis for 10 to 20 years may elect to have a liver biopsy performed in order to evaluate liver damage and establish a baseline histological profile. This procedure may be repeated every five years or so.

Q: What do you think about alpha-interferon (IFN)?

A: IFN is not an ideal therapy. Here are my reasons:

1. IFN has many side effects and a very low rate (15-20%) of therapeutic efficacy.

2. The advisory committee of the FDA, in desperation, recommended IFN. As Dr. Groopman, chair of the committee, wrote in "The Shadow Epidemic" (May 11, 1998, *The New Yorker*): "Back in 1991, when our advisory committee to the FDA voted to approve the drug (IFN), we had to acknowledge that there was no evidence that IFN treatment would save lives, but we were aware of the lack of any alternative, and of the desperate need of hepatitis C patients for relief....Seven years later, the options for treatment have barely changed."

3. IFN is one of many cytokines secreted by the cells of the immune system. These cytokines work in a balanced manner to keep the immune system functioning well. Introduction of millions of units of IFN inevitably disturbs immune function and causes immune disorders.

4. IFN treatment attempts only to eliminate the virus and does not address the complicated problems of liver diseases caused by viral hepatitis.

5. IFN itself is an antigen, and eventually the body will produce an antibody to it. The anti-IFN antibody can neutralize IFN and make it less effective. Moreover, with long-term use of IFN, HCV will undergo heightened mutation, creating new forms of the virus that may become IFN-resistant.

Q: Would the herbs in your protocol benefit someone taking IFN?

A: I have treated a few patients who were taking IFN as well as herbal remedies. They told me that they felt better and were experiencing fewer side effects of IFN while taking the herbs. More such cases are needed before we can give an evaluation of the blending of these two treatment regimens. As it is now, with so few of our patients using both IFN and the herbal formulas, it is very difficult for me to say whether the treatments are synergistic (helping each other) or antagonistic (working against each other). I can say, however, that no serious adverse reactions have been observed.

What I believe may be beneficial is to use a small dose of IFN (to avoid its side effects) for its antiviral effects and concurrently administer the herbal protocol to protect and heal the liver.

Q: What is your opinion of ribavirin?

A: Ribavirin was developed in the late 1980s and, when used alone for HCV, it produced poor results. Ribavirin is a nucleoside analogue that interferes with the HCV's RNA replication. This mechanism also interferes with DNA and RNA metabolism, thus it can alter genetic information in the cell and cause birth defects. Its chemical features are similar to AZT, used to treat HIV infection. I have worked with many HIV/AIDS patients and have seen that nucleoside analogues are toxic and can damage the liver. When used in combination treatment for HIV, common side effects of these nucleoside analogues are liver damage, elevated liver enzyme levels, jaundice, and fat deposits in the liver and abdomen. Besides, ribavirin has hemolytic (damages red blood cells) effects, which cause anemia.

Q: What do you think about Rebetron, the combination of IFN and ribavirin?

A: As a new combination therapy, the FDA had recently approved Rebetron. Reportedly, in clinical trials, the combination therapy had about a 50% sustained HCV suppression after the therapy stopped. However, every new treatment has a learning curve and we need time to evaluate its efficacy and side effects. It is too early to say whether this is a good combination. Nucleoside analogue is chemotherapy and it is hard on the liver. The side effects of Rebetron can be severe. In addition to the IFN side effects mentioned above, ribavirin may produce severe anemia that can lead to a heart attack or stroke in people with risk factors. Psychiatric problems have also been reported.

Q: Should I follow a special diet or avoid certain foods?

A: Yes, a proper diet can help by:

1. Improving metabolism of the liver and supporting metabolism of other organs and tissues,

2. Promoting repair and regeneration of liver cells,

3. Enhancing detoxification of the liver to reduce toxin accumulation and promoting decomposition and elimination of toxins,

4. Enhancing immunity,

5. Promoting storage and transportation of nutrients in the liver, and

6. Preventing dystrophic liver damage and nutritional deficiency secondary to the liver disease.

To accomplish the above, follow these dietary principles:

1. Consume sufficient daily protein, calculated in grams by dividing your body weight in pounds by 2. If your body weight is 150 pounds, for example, your daily protein requirement is 75 grams. It's best to get most of your protein from plant sources, such as tofu and beans, though some white meat is fine too. Only after liver disease has advanced to the later de-compensated stages should protein intake be limited.

2. If you are not overweight, consume sufficient daily calories, calculated by multiplying your body weight in pounds by 15. A 150-pound person, for example, would need 2,250 (150 x 15 = 2,250) calories per day.

3. Take vitamins and multi-vitamins in accordance with Dr. Andrew Weil's standard antioxidant formula: 1,000-2,000mg vitamin C and 25,000 IU mixed carotenoids at breakfast; 400-800 IU vitamin E and 200mcg selenium at lunch; and 1,000-2,000 vitamin C at dinner. Be careful not to take too much vitamin A (not more than 25,000 IU), since an overdose is toxic to the liver.

4. Strictly avoid all alcohol and tobacco. Alcohol is toxic to the liver and can accelerate liver disease, while smoking takes a major toll on the immune system.

5. Drink plenty of water. Flushing your kidneys with good-quality water (six to eight glasses a day) will allow your body's purification system to do its job and alleviate some of the workload of detoxification from the liver.

6. Avoid all drugs, whether prescribed, over-the-counter, or illegal. Since the liver metabolizes most drugs, even common painkillers such as acetaminophen, when combined with alcohol, can cause severe liver damage. If you're

taking prescription drugs, ask your doctor whether you truly need to stay on them. For liver disease, the principle is to take as few medications as possible. This principle applies to herbs as well—more is not better.

Q: What exercise do you recommend?

A: Exercise helps maintain general health. For people with chronic hepatitis, exercise should be gentle. Since the liver is the major source of energy for physical exercise, strenuous exercise can tax the liver. During exercise, blood supply to the liver is reduced. One of the best exercises for chronic hepatitis patients is walking. I advise my patients to reduce the amount and intensity of their exercise to 70% of their capability. Do not exercise to the point of fatigue.

One of my patients was feeling so well after her liver function normalized, she swam an hour a day for several weeks, after which her ALT elevated again. So don't strain yourself. Moderation is the key.

Q: Do I need plenty of rest?

A: Sufficient rest is very important. Don't work long hours, day after day. The liver is the major powerhouse of the body. All your energy for work and play comes from the liver. So set aside some time every day for qi-gong, meditation, or simply doing nothing.

6

Case Studies — Patient Stories

In this section I will tell you the stories of some of my patients. Their names have been changed, but their stories are real. You will see how my treatments have changed their lives. People may say that these are only anecdotes, but I would rather call them uncontrolled clinical outcome observations or case studies. Double-blind, placebo-controlled, randomized tests are important to evaluate a drug, but for an individual patient, a good clinical outcome is the most important thing. The majority of my patients have seen clinical outcomes similar to those of the following patients.

Linda S

Linda S, 46, was diagnosed with hepatitis C in July of 1996. Her biopsy showed that the disease was already at stage 4— the beginning of cirrhosis. Her ALT was 85 and her AST was 68. A viral load test with PCR in August 1997 found 18 million copies of HCV per milliliter of blood (quite a high level). By early February 1998, her ALT shot up to 386 and her AST was 213. She tried a vegetarian diet, weekly autohemotherapy (using one's own blood to treat oneself), ozone treatments, and a multitude of supplements. None of them helped. She was suffering arthritic pain, flu-like symptoms, brain fog, diarrhea, and digestion problems. She was desperate.

A friend of hers recommended Chinese medicine and gave her my name and phone number. She came to see me on February 6, 1998. I diagnosed her with chronic active hepatitis C with many auto-immune manifestations. She started to use Hepa Formula No. 2, Glycyrrhizin Capsule, Ligustrin Capsule, AI Capsule No. 3, and Circulation Tablet No. 1. Within three months, her blood was re-tested: ALT went from 386 to 49 (normal ranging 5 to 40), AST went from 213 to 44 (normal ranging from 5 to 40), and all the negative symptoms related to HCV disappeared. At present, she has more energy than she has had in years, and she is optimistic about living a long and healthy life. She accepted a position as dean of a New York City college. Here is Linda S's story in her own words.

My Story, by Linda S

I first noticed symptoms of fatigue in the fall of '93. In the preceding year my mentor passed away, my first book was published by a major publisher, I produced a successful show, my husband decided to change his career, and we saw our youngest son through four major eye surgeries. I consulted my physician, who concluded, without taking a blood test, "Your fatigue is from stress and depression. See a therapist."

I did. My psychiatrist prescribed an anti-depressant that took away the fatigue but brought on a whole range of other undesirable symptoms. I was switched to Ritalin because my con-

centration was minimal and the fatigue was increasing. "Typical adult attention deficit," she said. Soon I stopped eating, became faint and nauseous, and had constant diarrhea. I assumed these were side effects of the Ritalin.

In 1997, I had a general check-up with a physician who, after hearing my symptoms, insisted I take a blood test. I learned I had hepatitis C, stage 4, the beginnings of cirrhosis. My AST was 85 and my ALT was 68. I realized then that the fatigue I had experienced four years earlier was the first signal that I was ill, not a signal that I was depressed or stressed-out. Apparently two physicians had misdiagnosed my health problem for four years.

I researched interferon and realized it was not something I wanted to take. I changed my diet, took mega-supplements, and did ozone therapy for 18 months. First I got better, then I got worse. My AST and ALT levels rose to the 300s for the first time, my body always ached, I couldn't concentrate, I was scared and feeling very, very sick. Someone I befriended on the Internet suggested I contact Dr. Zhang. "Hey, you're desperate. Take a chance with Chinese medicine. What have you got to lose?" he e-mailed me one day.

I'm glad to say I took his suggestion. In early 1998 I contacted Dr. Zhang, and within six weeks of taking the herbs my ALT and AST levels were nearly normalized. Now, one and a half years later, I enjoy a completely normal life. I returned to full-time work as a college professor, I am working on a second book, I drive my two sons to all their hockey games, and I still have the energy to party with my husband on Saturday night! Thank you, Dr. Zhang!

Joanne M.

Joanne M, 63, came to my seminar on "Treating Viral Hepatitis With Modern Chinese Medicine" in Irvine, California, on May 8, 1999, with her husband, a retired physician. They were curious about what I was going to say. After a four-hour seminar, she and her husband were convinced and decided to use my protocol. She wrote: "I learned more from you in the four-hour seminar than I have in the past five years. I want to thank you so much. My husband is a retired M.D. and wants me to follow your program." Her primary care physician, Dr. Marek Z, is also willing to work with me to monitor her progress during the herbal treatments. She said, "One thing I will always be grateful to Dr. Marek Z for is that he urged me not to take interferon. It really didn't take urging because I have talked to people taking that treatment and they are all ill." After a little more than two months of taking my herbal treatments, she came to New York with her daughter to see me in my office.

My Story, by Joanne M

In 1994, during the course of a physical exam, I had routine lab work performed and my liver function tests were found to be abnormal. Further studies revealed that I tested positive for hepatitis C. I never had any symptoms. I could not imagine when I had contracted the disease, but I was thought to have had it for 20 to 30 years. Referral was made to a hepatologist, who recommended that I have interferon therapy, in spite of the fact that it was definitely contraindicated in my case because of coexisting thrombocytopenia (low platelet count) and anemia. I talked with several people who had received interferon therapy and who were constantly ill from the moment they started treatment until they stopped and were no better after treatment than before. Everyone I spoke to was advised to repeat the interferon therapy when it was found that the liver function tests elevated after the first course of treatment. Many refused the second course of therapy because it made them so ill. I decided not to take the recommended interferon treatment.

During the next few years, I felt relatively well, although I frequently had to take afternoon naps. There was very little change in my lab work, including LFTs (liver function tests).

Late in 1998, I began experiencing increasing fatigue, generalized arthralgia (joint pain), weekly episodes of chills and fever, episodes of diarrhea, and general malaise. I found myself spending several days each week in bed. The pain in my joints was becoming harder to bear, and I was afraid to take any pain medication because of my failing liver. The chills and fever caused me to think and talk inappropriately. Sometimes I couldn't get out of bed for days. My laboratory tests were worsening. My family was worried about me because I was so sick and tired. I became depressed and didn't want to get out of bed or leave my room. I talked to my gastroenterologist about the depression and his answer was to put me on Prozac—something I didn't want. My primary care physician recommended in March 1999 that I be evaluated for a liver transplant and get my name on the liver transplant list at UCLA.

It was at this time that I read an article by Dr. Andrew Weil about Dr. Zhang, who was treating hepatitis C patients with herbal therapy and getting some very good results. I later attended a lecture given by Dr. Zhang and was very impressed by him and the work he was doing treating patients with HCV, HBV, and HIV. After hearing him speak, I decided to try his *herbal treatment. After only two weeks of herbal therapy, I began to feel better. I have now been on Dr. Zhang's herbal program for 10 weeks. My fatigue, arthralgia, episodic chills and fever, and diarrhea are gone, and my energy has returned. I have a general feeling of well being. My LFTs were repeated after being on this treatment for six weeks and all liver enzymes were improved. I was able to make a long-anticipated trip to New York City with my daughter and grandchildren. A year earlier, I could never have made this trip. My daughter felt I had more energy than she did. I am so grateful to Dr. Zhang.*

Joanne M is still feeling well, and her liver function is continuously improving. Her recent liver enzyme tests (July 1, 1999) showed that her ALT was 32, down from 190. This was the first normal reading since her diagnosis in 1994. Her ALT had been around 150 since 1994. Her AST was now 106, down from 230. Especially significant was that her AFP (alpha fetal protein) level started to come down. It had been around 180 (normal < 15) for more than four years, not a good sign, as this could indicate tumor growth. After taking the herbal remedies for six weeks, her AFP dropped from 177.3 to 120.4. I prescribed a special formula, R-6532, for treating AFP elevation.

Now she is on this formula and we expect more improvement. On October 6, 1999, she re-tested her blood chemistry and liver functions after five months on the herbal treatment. Her ALT was 29 and stayed in the normal range. Her bilirubin direct came down to 0.6 from 0.9, while bilirubin total came down from 2.3 to 1.4. Most importantly, her AFP reduced to 44.3 from 120.4. Two figures worsened: her AST increased from 106 to 156 and her AKP from 181 to 242. Overall, though, her condition was continuing to improv, as of this writing.

Judy C

Judy C, 33, contracted hepatitis B from her mother when she was born. Though she suffered from hepatitis B, rather than C, her case is included here to provide additional evidence of the efficacy of an herbal treatment for hepatitis.

When she came to see me on May 16, 1998, she wasn't able to work and was always tired. She had yellowish conjunctiva and light jaundice in her skin, her urine was the color of strong tea, and her stool was often clay-colored. She often experienced nausea and vomiting. She retained water and had obvious ankle edema. She complained of a constant dull pain in her liver area, and her stomach was distended. She suffered multiple joint pain and morning stiffness. Her skin was so itchy that she couldn't stop scratching.

Upon her initial visit, her ALT was 382, her AST was 208, her GGT was 89 (normal ranging from 5 to 80), and her AFP was 46.1 (normal<15). Her HBsAg (hepatitis B virus surface antigen) and HBeAg (hepatitis B virus e antigen) were positive. Her anti-HBs (hepatitis B virus surface antibody) and anti-HBe (hepatitis B virus e antibody) were both negative. Her liver enzyme levels had been elevated for more than 10 years.

After herbal treatment started, she monitored her LFTs every month. One month after the herbal therapy, her ALT dropped from 382 to 146, her AST rose to 283 from 208, and her GGT rose to 203 from 89. She had a mixed reaction in the first month, since GGT and AST relate more to chronic conditions (especially GGT, which indicates bile retention, consistent with her jaundice). I added Gall Formula No. 1 to facilitate bile secretion. One month later, on July 15, 1998, her ALT dropped to 62, AST decreased to 71, and GGT dropped to 100. At this time, her anti-HBe became positive and her HBeAg turned negative. This was an important change, because HBeAg turning negative signals that HBV replication has dramatically reduced. HBeAb becoming positive means that the immune system has started to produce anti-HBV antibody and the patient is therefore less infectious to others. But the same test showed her AFP went up to 80.8. This caused her concern, so I prescribed a special formula coded R-6532 (used for preventing and treating tumors). After I added this formula to her hepatitis B protocol for one month, on August 12, 1998, her ALT and AST were found to have reduced to normal levels for the first time in 10 years—19 and 29, respectively. At the same time, her GGT dropped from 100 to 51—within the normal range. More importantly, her AFP dropped from 80.8 to 18.7. And two months later, on October 11, 1998, her ALT and AST dropped further to 14 and 22, and her AFP dropped down to 6.08.

As of this writing, her LFTs remain normal. Her jaundice is totally gone. Her overall health has greatly improved. The most recent blood work done on June 23, 1999, showed that her ALT was 8, her AST was 14, her GGT was 17, and her AFP was 3.50. She went back to work and is planning to have a baby.

Lorraine D

Lorraine D, 41, works for a large pharmaceutical company that produces alpha-interferon (IFN). She came to see me on May 26, 1998, for hepatitis C, after suffering a relapse from her IFN treatment.

She had been diagnosed with hepatitis C in 1997 and believes she might have contracted the virus seven years before through sexual contact.

Two months before her initial visit, in March 1998, she decided to stop a seven-month course of IFN treatment (August 1997 to March 1998). At that time, her liver function tests were normal: ALT was 16 and AST was 20. But the side effects of IFN were so severe she could not continue the treatment. Her platelet count was depleted to 29, a dangerously low level. She often had black and blue marks on her skin. Because of this, she was diagnosed as having idiopathic thrombocytopenic purpura (ITP), an auto-immune disease, and was given prednisone every day. Her thyroid gland function was also seriously disturbed. Her TSH was 0.03 (normal range 0.35-5.50) and her T4 (thyroxine) was 15.5 (normal range 4.5-12). She was given Synthroid to correct the thyroid function.

Prednisone treatment helped the platelet count to increase to 86 in two months, but carried with it the risk of triggering a relapse of the liver inflammation. On May 11, 1998, her ALT went up to 112 and AST to 72. Right before she came to see me, a blood test showed that her liver enzyme levels were still elevated: ALT was 98, AST was 54, and GGT was 77, with a very high viral load of 27million/ml. The liver inflammation relapsed only two months after the IFN treatment stopped, and the viral load was much higher than before the IFN treatments. The disease had come back. Lorraine was very tired and had pain in her liver area and joints, dark urine, and occasional diarrhea with pale stool. Her skin and conjunctiva were yellowish. In addition, she had a pituitary tumor as an underlying condition, which made her situation very complicated. Her conventional doctor suggested Rebetron (IFN plus ribavirin), but she refused. She definitely didn't want to go back to IFN treatment, but she didn't know where to go or what approach to use. She felt lost.

At this point, a friend told her the story of Joseph V's successful treatment with my herbal remedies (see Chapter 1). At the same time, she read Dr. Andrew Weil's recommendation of my herbal treatments for viral hepatitis in his newsletter *Self Healing*. Lorraine decided to try my approach.

She came to see me on May 26, 1998. To treat such a complicated case, I decided first to focus on her liver inflammation. Her ITP and thyroid gland dysfunction showed that her liver inflammation had auto-immunity involvement. I emphasized anti-auto-immune-reaction therapy. She began taking Hepa Formula No. 2, Glycyrrhizin Capsule, Ligustrin Capsule, AI Capsule No. 3, Circulation Tablet No. 1, and Formula R6379 (the latter of which is specifically for hypothyroidism). One month after taking these herbal remedies, on June 27, 1998, her blood tests showed that all her liver enzyme levels had normalized, ALT had dropped to 12, AST was down to 19, and GGT was 41. Her platelet count had normalized at 152. At the same time, her TSH (1.34) and T4 (10.5) also showed normal values. She was ecstatic, since the treatment had killed three birds with one stone, normalizing all her ITP and ridding her of hypothyroidism and liver inflammation in only one month.

Since then, her liver enzyme levels have been normal, except once in reaction to a drug treatment for edema in her ankle, when her ALT, AST, and GGT temporarily rose to 66, 67, and 103, respectively, in October 1998. By the next month, they were normal again. The most recent readings, taken on September 23, 1999, showed her ALT and AST were 8 and 25, respectively, and her GGT was 49, with a viral load of 285,000 (down from 27 million/ml). Her platelet count was 244, and thyroid functions were normal. Now she is on a maintenance protocol. All her symptoms are gone. As a by-product of this treatment, her pap smear test done on July 9, 1999, showed no displasia, which had always been positive in previous tests. This means that her immune system function was greatly strengthened by the herbal hepatitis protocol.

John P

John P, 66, was a senior editor of a nationally known business magazine. He was referred to me by Dr. Andrew Weil's integrative medicine project at the University of Arizona. John became infected with the HCV through a blood transfusion during surgery in June 1983. John lives in Dallas, though he moved to New York for a few months so I could treat him. I first saw him on September 5, 1998. His disease was in a very advanced decompensation stage with ascites in the stomach and edema in the ankles and legs. His spleen was greatly enlarged—the size of a small watermelon. His liver enzyme levels had continued to rise since his diagnosis in 1983. His platelet count was lower than 50, and he already had varices in his esophagus and stomach. His prothrombine time was prolonged. He had an episode of intestinal bleeding that required hospitalization. His first liver biopsy in 1990 found early cirrhosis. From 1992 on, he had interferon treatments on and off without success. He was a regular drinker until he finally stopped in 1995. He was very weak and thin with a grayish complexion. He also suffered memory loss and occasional disorientation. His hands had very obvious liver palms, and spider moles were visible on his chest. Endoscopy found varicose veins in his stomach wall. He had been on the liver transplant list, but because his cardiomyopathy (a disease of the heart muscle) caused second-to third-degree heart failure (he had only 25% of his heart function left), he could not tolerate the transplant surgery. He had arrhythmia with frequent premature heartbeats. He was looking into a dual organ transplant—the liver and heart at the same time. But his age (65) and poor health prevented him from undergoing such large-scale surgery. In addition, he also had severe psoriasis in his legs and psoriatic arthritis pain. A diabetic, John's blood sugar level was above 190 (normal range 90-120). He was truly desperate.

When he came to my office, I was very hesitant to take him as a patient. His condition was beyond or at the edge of my ability to take care of him as an outpatient. Because he was referred by Dr. Andrew Weil's office and because he had moved from so far from home to see me, I decided to try my best. At the same time, I cautioned him and his wife that if any bleeding, black stool, or disorientation occurred, he was to rush to a hospital emergency room.

Before he came to see me, his liver function tests were: ALT, 78; AST, 212; GGT, 258; and platelet count, 40.

AST/ALT was greater than 2.7. I started with small doses and used many preventive measures, especially herbal remedies, to prevent bleeding. I advised him to limit his salt and protein intake.

I prescribed Hepa Formula No. 3, Gall Formula No. 1, Ligustrin Capsule, AI Capsule No. 3, Circulation Tablet No.1, Cordyceps Capsule, and a topical ointment for psoriasis—all in half doses. I gave him Yunnan Pai Yao Capsule as a preventative for possible bleeding. At the same time, I treated him with acupuncture.

He responded very well to treatment. One week later, he told me that he had taken a walk along the beach—something he hadn't been able to do for long time. He had more energy and felt more alert. His psoriasis was improving, and some lesions had disappeared. His long-term diarrhea and loose stool stopped. His grayish complexion improved and he could sleep better. The frequency of his premature heartbeat was reduced. But his urine still had the color of strong tea and his spleen and liver areas were very uncomfortable with a dull pain. He felt that this was because his swollen liver and spleen had begun to shrink. After only one week, he was encouraged by these improvements.

Two weeks later, his spleen continued to shrink and returned above the navel. His ascites started to reduce, and his liver pain became rare and mild. His complexion improved further and his psoriasis lesions almost disappeared. I started him on full doses of all the herbs.

Forty days after he started the herbal treatments, his blood tests showed ALT had reduced from 78 to 61, AST from 212 to 124, and GGT from 258 to 116. His bilirubin total, however, had increased from 1.2 to 2.2, his platelet count had reduced from 40 to 33, and his blood sugar level was 212. So his test results were a mixed bag. But, more important to John than lab results, his subjective symptoms had all improved. Physically, his spleen continued to shrink, and the liver area pain became very rare. His psoriasis lesions were almost gone and his psoriatic arthritis pain disappeared. One new problem was that his elevated blood sugar level caused peripheral neuropathy and made his ankles swell up and his legs become weak and numb. I continued his protocol and added Corydalin Tablet (an extract from *Corydalis yanhusao Rhizoma*) to deal with his peripheral neuropathy.

He could only stay in New York for about two months; on October 29, 1998, he visited my office for the last time. When I palpated his spleen, it had shrunk to a grapefruit size and his ascites in the stomach had disappeared. He went back to Dallas, taking enough herbs with him to continue the herbal treatment. On December 8, 1998, his lab tests showed ALT was 54, AST was 140, bilirubin direct 0.5, bilirubin total 1.6, and platelets 43. His condition was stable and his heart function had recovered from degree II heart failure. His prothrombin time (14.5 seconds) and PTT (37.3 seconds) were both normalized. Although he was still in an advanced cirrhotic condition, he was much better than before the treatment. He was even able to travel to California to have Christmas with his daughter's family.

In the summer of 1999, further tests found cancer in his liver. John died in July 1999.

John's was not a typical outpatient case, though John's story illustrates that my herbal treatment can help improve overall health, quality of life, and life span of patients in advanced stages of the disease. For those awaiting liver transplantation, this treatment can help extend their waiting time and help them to be better prepared to undergo this serious surgery.

Michael M

Michael M, 44, a computer expert from Akron, Ohio, heard about my herbal treatment for hepatitis C and called for a phone consultation. I suggested he take Group I herbs (Hepa Formula No. 2, Glycyrrhizin Capsule, Ligustrin Capsule, and Circulation Tablet No. 1). Six months later, he mailed me a set of beautiful computer graphics that showed how his condition had improved (see below).

HCV RNA PCR Quantitative (Viral Load)

Reference Range 0-200

November	1998	N/A
December	1998	790,947
---------- Began treatment January 11, 1999 --------		
March	1999	159,120
May	1999	5,609
July	1999	241

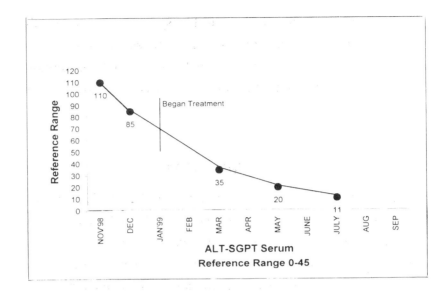

ALT-SGPT Serum
Reference Range 0-45

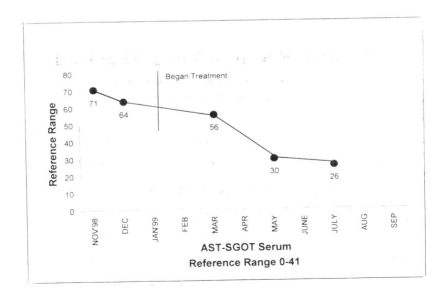

AST-SGOT Serum
Reference Range 0-41

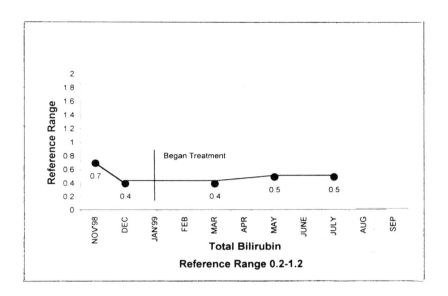

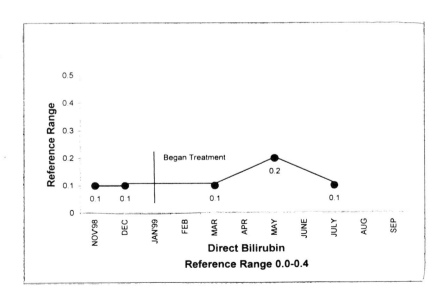

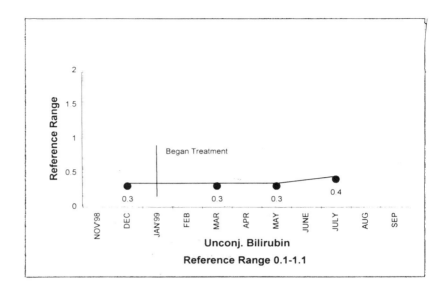

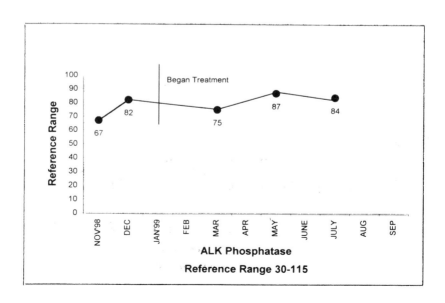

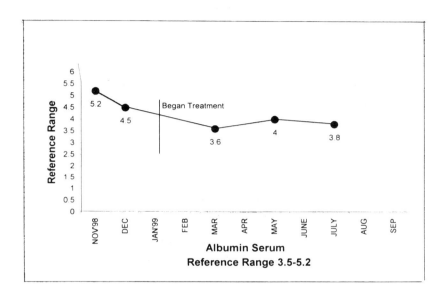

Albumin Serum
Reference Range 3.5-5.2

Phone consultation is one way I have helped those who can't come to New York. I prefer to work over the phone with those who have mild or common symptoms. For those suffering from severe complications and symptoms, a one-on-one consultation is necessary.

APPENDIX

The Efficacy of Zhang's Chinese Herbal Protocol in Treating Hepatitis C: A Retrospective Analysis of its Clinical Practice

Abstract

Objective: To observe the therapeutic efficacy of Zhang's Chinese Herbal Protocol (ZCHP) in treating chronic viral hepatitis C.

Method: A retrospective analysis of the changes of liver enzyme ALT level of patients treated with ZCHP.

Results: In a total of 75 cases with complete liver function test (LFTs) records, the average level of ALT before and after the treatment were, respectively, 128.441 ± 113.75 and 47.29 ± 41.60. The difference was 81.15 ± 114.54, a very significant improvement of ALT level ($p < 0.001$). Among these patients, 77% had their ALT level normalized and 93% improved. AST and viral load were reduced, though with no statistical significance. Subjective symptoms improved with every patient.

Conclusion: Zhang's Chinese Herbal Protocol provides an effective alternative treatment for chronic hepatitis C.

Key words: Chinese medicine, hepatitis C, ALT, AST, HCV viral load

In April 1998, Dr. Andrew Weil published the article "Natural Help for Hepatitis C" in his newsletter *Self Healing*.[1] In the article, Zhang's Chinese Herbal Protocol (ZCHP) was mentioned as an alternative treatment for hepatitis C (Hep C). As a result, an overwhelming number of patients responded and sought help from our clinic. Since then, we have focused our clinical and research work on treating chronic Hep C with modern Chinese herbal medicine. We are currently treating more than 600 chronic viral hepatitis patients; about half of them are outpatients and half are consulting with us. The vast majority of them have responded very well. In order to see how statistically significant the efficacy of this protocol is, we made a retrospective analysis of its clinical outcome. This article reports the results of this analysis.

Clinical Data

Among the 300+ patients who visited our office and have filed clinical data in our office, 188 of them have partial LFTs records, 180 have pre-treatment records, and 86 have post-treatment records. Only 75 patients have both pre- and post-treatment LFTs records. These 75 cases were used for this retrospective analysis. We used their pre- and post-treatment LFTs records, especially the ALT level, as a main criterion to evaluate the therapeutic efficacy of ZCHP. The conventional medical doctors of these patients had already made the diagnosis of chronic viral hepatitis before they came to visit us. Among these patients, 27 were female and 48 are male. They were all in the chronic stage of the disease, and infection durations were estimated to be between 20 and 30 years. Because most patients could not determine the exact date of infection, infection durations could not be accurately measured. Only seven cases had HCV genotype records: five of genotype 1a and two of 1b. Most of these patients had taken ZCHP for a period of three to six months, and a few had used the treatment for more than a year. They visited our office once a month or once every other month, and had their LFTs done in two-to-three-month intervals.

The Herbal Protocol

The herbal remedies we use in treating viral hepatitis consist of single herbs and herbal formulas. All these products are made from herbal extracts and active ingredients. The phytopharmacology of these active ingredients have all been well studied. The clinical applications are based on their pharmacology, and on their respective usage in Traditional Chinese Medicine (TCM). With the development of new extraction and purification techniques, we can now use more potent forms of these herbal remedies, and they can be taken in smaller doses. These herbal products are semi-standardized and their therapeutic actions are predictable and can be replicated. This author personally developed ZCHP. The herbal products are manufactured by Sun Ten Laboratories and distributed by HepaPro Corporation in California, USA. The following herbal remedies are used in the basic regimens of ZCHP:

1. Hepa Formula No. 2, (consists of *Schizandrae Fructus, Artemisiae capillaris Herba, Alismatis Rhizoma, Polyporus, Poria, Atractylodes Rhizoma, Cinnamomi Ramulus, Citri Pericarpium, Magnoliae Cortex, Zingiberis Rhizoma,* and *Glycyrrhizae Radix*). The active ingredients of *Schizandrae*: Schizandrin B and C are the main ingredients. Dosage: 500mg per capsule. Take 2 capsules 3 times a day.

2. Glycyrrhizin (GL) Capsule: Its main ingredient is a potassium salt of glycyrrhizic acid. Dosage: Each capsule contains 150mg of GL. Take 1 capsule, twice a day.

3. Ligustrin Capsule: Its main ingredient is oleanolic acid. Dosage: Each capsule contains 40mg of olenolic acid. Take 1 capsule, 3 times a day.

4. Circulation No. 1 Tablet consists of *Carthami Flos, Persicae Semen, Angelicae Radix, Cnidii Rhizoma, Rehmanniae Radix, Paeoniae rubra Radix, Achyranthis Radix, Citri aurantii Fructus, Bupleuri Radix, Glycyrrhizae Radix, Platycodi Radix.* Dosage: 500mg per tablet. Take 4 tablets, 3 times a day.

These four herbal remedies were combined as Group I, which was used by every patient except those with hypertension. For the latter, GL could not be used, therefore Group II was prescribed, which consists of Hepa Formula No. 2, Ligustrin and Circulation No. 1. For those with individual symptoms and complications, other herbal remedies were added to treat specific conditions. For manifestations of jaundice, elevation of bilirubin, cholangitis, and cholelithiasis (gallstone), Gall No. 1 Tablet was added. In the case of autoimmune manifestations (joint pain, skin rashes, vasculitis, etc.), AI#3 Capsule was added. For insomnia, HerbSom Capsule was used. For severe fatigue, Cordyceps Capsule was used.

We strongly suggested that patients check their LFTs every two to three months after taking the herbs. If their LFT readings were normal for three consecutive times within one year, and each reading was two to three months apart, then we would switch them to the maintenance protocol to sustain long-term results.

Results of Clinical Data Analysis

The ALT, AST, GGT, AKP, bilirubin, and HCV RNA PCR of the 75 patients were collected. The average and standard deviations of pre- and post-treatment figures of ALT and AST were calculated. Statistically significant t-test for related population was used to test the confidence limit. Results are listed in the following table.

	Pre-treatment	Post-treatment	Improvement	Normalized	Improved
ALT	128 44 ± 113.75	47.29 ± 41.60	81.15 ± 114.54*	77% (57/75)	93% (69/75)
AST	86.69 ± 66.08	79.34 ± 47.90	7.35 ± 66.46**	25% (19/75)	51% (38/75)

N = 75   * P < 0.001   **P < 0.4

In 75 cases with complete ALT records, the average readings of ALT before and after treatment were 128.44±113.75 and 47.29±41.60, respectively. The difference was 81.15± 114.54, a very significant improvement of ALT level (P<0.001). Among these patients, 57/75 (77%) had their ALT level normalized and 69/75 (93%) improved. Because the normal range of ALT varies in different labs (most labs set their normal range from 5 to 40), when a patient's ALT level was less than 40, we considered it to be within normal range. For those labs that have higher ranges, we used their range.

AST changes were also calculated. The average readings of AST before and after treatment were 86.69±66.08 and 79.34 ±47.90, respectively. The difference was 7.35±66.46, which was not statistically significant (P<0.4). Compared with pretreatment levels, 38 patients (51%) improved, and among them, 19 (25%) were normalized. Compared with the changes in ALT levels, AST levels were not as responsive to ZCHP.

Only 18 cases had HCV RNA PCR quantitative (viral load) records before treatment, and the average number was 2,085,800/ml. Only 16 people had viral load figures after treatment, average of 1,523,900/ml. We did not do a statistical test for viral load, because ZCHP was not particularly designed to be anti-viral. The reduction of the viral load might be the result of the restoration of liver functions and overall health. Subjective symptoms improved in all 75 patients. Patients reported that they received a sensation of well being and experienced much less fatigue. Pain and discomfort within the liver area were relieved in about three to six weeks. Joint pain and muscle aches were reduced in a few weeks. Dark urine and pale stool disappeared in a few weeks. Objective physical signs, such as yellowish skin and conjunctiva, spider mole, and liver palm, also became less pronounced and disappeared in many cases.

Case Study

Lorraine D, age 41, first visited our office on May 26, 1998, for hepatitis C after suffering a relapse from interferon (IFN) treatment. She had been diagnosed in 1997, and she might have contracted the infection seven years ago. She works for a large pharmaceutical company, which produces alpha-interferon.

In March 1998, she stopped a seven-month course of interferon treatment (August 1997 to March 1998). At the end of the treatment, her LFTs readings were normal, ALT was 16 and AST was 20. However, the side effects of IFN were too severe and she had to stop the treatment. Her platelet count was depleted to 29, a dangerously low level. She often had black and blue marks on her skin, and was also diagnosed with idiopathic thrombocytopenic purpura (ITP), an autoimmune disease. She was given prednisone every day. Her thyroid gland functions were also seriously disturbed. Her TSH was 0.03 (normal range 0.35-5.50) and her T4 was 15.5 (normal 4.5-12). She was given Syntharoid to correct the thyroid function. Prednisone treatment helped to increase her platelet count to 86 in two months, but it triggered a relapse of liver inflammation. On May 11, 1998, her ALT was tested to be 112 and AST 72. Immediately prior to her visit to our clinic, her blood test showed that her liver enzyme levels were still elevated. ALT was 98, AST was 54, and GGT was 77 with a very high viral load of 27million/ml. Liver inflammation relapsed two months after the IFN treatment, and viral load rose and became much higher than before the IFN treatments. At the same time, she was experiencing much fatigue, had much pain in her liver area and joints, dark urine, and occasional had diarrhea with pale stool. Her skin and conjunctiva were yellowish. In addition, she had a pituitary tumor as an underlying condition, which further complicated her situation. Her conventional doctor suggested using Rebetron, but she declined. At that time she read Dr. Andrew Weil's recommendation of the herbal treatments for viral hepatitis of Zhang's Clinic, and decided to give it a try.

Her ITP and hypothyroidism indicated that her liver inflammation was mainly caused by autoimmune reactions. Therefore, while treating her liver inflammation, we also emphasized anti-autoimmune therapy. The treatment protocol consisted of Hepa Formula No. 2, Glycyrrhizin Capsule, Ligustrin Capsule,

Circulation No. 1 Tablet, AI #3 Capsule, and Formula R6379 (used to treat hypothyroidism). One month after taking these herbal remedies, on June 27, 1998, her blood tests showed that all her liver enzyme levels had become normal, ALT dropped to 12, AST to 19, and GGT to 41. Her platelet count normalized at 152. At the same time, her TSH (1.34) and T4 (10.5) also normalized. The treatment had normalized her ITP, hypothyroidism, and liver inflammation within one month, and all of her previous symptoms were gone.

In tracing her post-treatment condition, we found that her liver enzyme levels have been normal ever since, with only one exception, which was in reaction to a drug treatment for edema in her ankle, when her ALT, AST, and GGT temporarily rose to 66, 67, and 103, respectively, in October 1998. By the next month, however, her enzyme levels returned to normal again. A blood test on September 23, 1999, showed that her ALT and AST were 8 and 25, GGT was 49, and viral load was 285,000/ml (down from 27 million/ml). Her platelets were 244, and thyroid functions were normal. She is currently using the maintenance protocol.

Another positive result was that her PAP smear done on July 9, 1999, showed no displasia, which had always been positive in previous tests. This demonstrates that her immune functions have been strengthened by the herbal protocol. When her immunity and health improved, the viral load dropped dramatically. From this case, we can see that ZCHP is a comprehensive approach that can help control liver inflammation and improve overall health.

Discussion

This is a preliminary retrospective analysis of the clinical outcome of the ZCHP. In the absence of a control group and randomization, there might be some biases. Zhang's Clinic is an alternative healthcare clinic, and we rely on our patients' conventional doctors to monitor the progress of their respective conditions during the herbal treatment. As a result, we could only recommend, but could not require, patients to have their laboratory tests done regularly. Thus, it is difficult for every patient to have complete liver function tests (LFTs) records. In addition, we have no control over patients taking other supplements and medications. In cases where conventional doctors use antibiotics to treat infections such as sinusitis and bronchitis, these antibiotics can cause fluctuations in liver enzyme levels. In spite of these uncertainties, however, we were still able to achieve significant improvements in ALT levels. To monitor the progression of hepatitis C, ALT is not as direct an indicator as is a biopsy. But because a biopsy is an invasive procedure, many patients tend to avoid it. As an alternative, ALT is an important monitoring method.[2] After treatment with continuous normal ALT, liver inflammation can be considered under control. Control of the inflammation is key to halting the progression of liver disease and to suspending development of cirrhosis.

One important phenomenon in this treatment is that along with the improvement in LFT readings, patients became much healthier. This is quite different from the conventional treatment with IFN and Rebetron, which often make patients sicker while LFT figures are improving in responders. This difference is due to the fact that the herbal remedies in ZCHP are liver-function-restoring and virtually non-toxic, and they are beneficial to the overall health of the human body.

This retrospective analysis is a meaningful first step, which indicates that a well-designed double-blind, placebo-controlled, and randomized trial to further test ZCHP's efficacy is worthwhile. The semi-standardization of the herbal remedies used in ZCHP has created a better treatment for that kind of trial than using raw Chinese herbs.

The most common criticism of herbal medicine is that herbs are unstable in respect to their active essence, since species, collecting seasons, and production sites are likely to vary. Furthermore, the method of preparation (drying, steaming, and decocting) may dilute the active essence of the herbs. Finally, it is objected that herbal medicines are inconvenient to prepare for ingestion. Variables can be reconciled through scientific preparation procedures to achieve a consistent pharmacological effect, and extracts can be concentrated to the point that the daily dosage is small and requires no special preparation. ZCHP has already utilized such preparation methods and is able to avoid these variations.

References

1. Andrew Weil, "Natural Help for Hepatitis," *Dr. Andrew Weil's Self Healing*, April 1998, pp. 1, 6-7.

2. "Managing Hepatitis C: The NIH Consensus Statement—Implications and Issues" (revised draft), 3/27/97.

Glossary

Acupuncture

A traditional Chinese medical therapy involving insertion of fine needles into particular points on the body that correspond to specific organ systems.

Acute hepatitis

Inflammation of the liver of less than six months' duration.

AKP or ALP

Alkaline phosphatase, a liver and bone enzyme that can be measured in the bloodstream. It increases during chronic hepatitis, especially when there is an intra-liver blockage of bile secretion.

Albumin

A serum protein synthesized in the liver, used as an indicator of liver protein synthetic function.

ALT (SGPT)

Alanine aminotransferase, which previously was termed serum glutamic-pyruvic transaminase. A liver enzyme that can be measured in the bloodstream. It is an important lab marker for liver inflammation and liver cell damage.

Antibody

A protein released by the immune system that can fight a specific antigen.

Antigen

A substance that can cause immune reactions and antibody production.

Ascites

Accumulation of fluid within the abdomen. In liver disease, it is an indicator that the disease has reached the decompensated stage.

AST (SGOT)

Aspartate aminotransferase, which was previously termed serum glutamic-oxaloacetic transaminase. A liver enzyme that can be measured in the bloodstream. It is a lab marker for liver inflammation and liver cell damage. Since the majority of AST is in the heart, it is less specific than ALT in monitoring liver inflammation.

Autoimmunity

An immune reaction to one's own tissues.

Bilirubin

A waste product of hemoglobin metabolism that is normally eliminated from the body through bile secretion. Retention of bilirubin can cause jaundice and promote fibrosis in the liver.

Biopsy

The surgical removal of a tissue sample from a living body for histological (microscopic) diagnostic tests.

Blood rheology

A study of the liquidity features of the blood.

Blood stagnancy

A traditional Chinese medicine term to describe the symptom pattern of dark tongue, dark lips, cold hands and feet, dark rings around the eyes, dry skin, and body aches. In chronic liver disease, blood stagnancy is common.

Cancer

Malignant tumor. Cancer cells are not well differentiated, proliferate rapidly, and can metastasize to other sites.

Chronic hepatitis

Liver inflammation lasting more than six months that becomes a persistent or recurring liver disease.

Circulatory immune complex (CIC)

A virus that stimulates the body to produce antibodies to form an antibody-antigen complex that circulates in the bloodstream. When it deposits in the blood vessels of the liver, joints, and kidneys, it can cause inflammationo.

Cirrhosis

A sign of stage 4 liver fibrosis. At this stage, normal liver tissue has been mostly replaced by scar tissue.

Cryoglobulinemia

A common complication of hepatitis C in which a cold-sensitive protein (cryoglobuline) circulates in the bloodstream.

Cytopathic

Causing direct destruction to cells.

Decompensated cirrhosis

The scarred liver associated with symptoms of ascites, variceal bleeding, and disorientation (encephalopathy).

Depression

A mental state characterized by disinterest in life, anxiety, guilt, and poor concentration that can lead to suicidal thinking. A common complication of chronic liver disease.

DNA

Deoxyribonucleic acid, which consists of four nucleotide building blocks strung together in chains of thousands of molecules. The carrier of genetic information of living things. Hepatitis B virus is an example of a DNA virus.

Edema

Body fluid accumulation in the soft tissues, particularly in the legs and ankles.

Encephalopathy

A complication of decompensated liver disease; the mental confusion caused by toxic metabolic waste accumulation in the brain.

Fibrosis

Scar tissue formation caused by persistent inflammation, which can result in cirrhosis in chronic liver disease.

Genotype

A virus strain with a distinct genetic makeup.

GGT (gamma-GTP or GGTP)

Gamma-glutamyl-transpeptidase; a liver enzyme that can be measured in the bloodstream; a lab marker for liver-inflammatory activities during chronic hepatitis.

Glycogen

Polymerized glucose stored in the liver when the blood sugar level rises after eating.

HCV

Hepatitis C virus; the causative factor of hepatitis C; an example of an RNA virus.

Hepatitis C

Liver inflammation caused by hepatitis C virus infection.

Hepatologist

Doctor specializing in liver disease.

Histology

The study of microscopic tissue and cell structure.

HIV

Human immunodeficiency virus; the causative factor of AIDS.

Immunopathic

Causing tissue and cell destruction due to inadequate immune reactions.

Interferons (IFNs)

A group of mediators that increase the resistance of cells to viral infection and act as cytokines. Has been synthesized and used to treat hepatitis C.

Jaundice

Yellowish color seen in the skin and conjunctiva (whites of the eye) as a result of bilirubin retention in the liver caused by liver inflammation or blockage of bile secretion.

Liver function tests (LFTs)

Tests of liver protein synthetic function (albumin), transaminases (liver enzymes, ALT, AST, GGT, etc.) and bilirubin levels. LFTs are lab markers of the severity of liver disease and can be a useful measure of the progression of liver damage.

Microcirculation

Blood circulation in the micro-capillaries. During chronic liver disease, microcirculation deteriorates in the liver and other parts of the body.

PCR

Polymerase chain reaction. A test used to detect extremely low quantities of DNA or RNA, useful as a diagnostic and monitoring parameter of anti-HCV treatment in hepatitis C patients. Qualitative HCV RNA PCR test establishes the HCV's existence in the blood. Reported as positive or negative result. Quantitative HCV RNA PCR test determines the amount of the HCV RNA in the blood. The FDA has not yet endorsed it as a diagnostic method.

Portal vein hypertension

Blood pressure increase in the portal vein caused by liver inflammation and fibrosis, which increase the resistance of the blood going into the liver; the main pathology of the advanced stage of chronic liver disease.

Rebetron

Combination of interferon and ribavirin; one of the conventional treatments for hepatitis C.

Ribavirin

A nucleoside analog used as an anti-viral drug that mimics one of the building blocks of RNA and DNA.

RNA

Ribonucleic acid. Consists of four nucleotide building blocks strung together in chains of thousands of molecules. HCV is an example of an RNA virus.

Varices

Distended blood vessels in the stomach and esophagus caused by hypertension in the portal vein.

Viral load

A measure of the number of viral particles in the bloodstream, which is usually measured by a quantitative PCR test.

Virus

A microscopic particle of nucleic acid and protein that, upon entering a living cell, can replicate itself by using the cell's metabolism.

Index

Abscess 85

Acetylcholine 65, 68

Acupuncture 5, 113

Acute hepatitis 19, 76

Adenovirus 565

AFP (alpha fetal protein) 106, 107, 108

AKP (alkaline phosphatase) 25, 37, 39, 55, 67, 106

AI Capsule No. 3 36, 64, 92, 102, 110, 113

Albumin 43, 80, 94

Allicin 42, 43, 82, 83

Allicin Capsule 42, 82, 83

Allicin Solution 83

Allitridi 82, 83

Aloe-emodin 86

Alpha-interferon 96, 109

ALT (SGPT) 4, 8, 13, 20, 21, 22-24, 31-33, 38, 39, 47, 48, 50, 51, 52, 54, 67, 73-76, 80, 89, 100-103, 106-114

AMA 20, 41

Ameba 82, 84, 85

ANA 20, 41

Analgesic 65, 70

Anemia 12, 98, 104

ANIT (alpha-naphthyl isothiocyanate) 67

Anorexia 20

Anti-cancer 52, 84, 86

Anti-depressant 102

Anti-fibrosis 39

Anti-HBe 107, 108

Anti-HBs 107

Anti-HBV 90, 108

Anti-HCV 18, 23

Anti-inflammatory 15, 25, 52, 53, 70, 73, 74, 80, 91

Anti-lipemic 54

Anti-lithiasis 55

Anti-neoplastic 70, 80

Anti-viral 15, 17, 21, 22, 23, 28, 52, 56, 57, 73, 77, 78, 84, 90, 91, 97

Antibacterial 65, 77, 78, 84, 86

Antioxidant 63, 71, 82, 99

Antipyretic 73

Anxiety 49, 72

Appetite 11, 21, 68

Arrhythmia 81, 85, 112

Arthralgia 105, 106

Arthritis 25, 35, 64, 65, 102, 112, 114

Ascites 38, 40, 43, 59, 61, 80, 93, 111, 113, 114

AST (SGOT) 4, 21-27, 29, 30, 32-44, 46-49, 51, 52, 56, 57, 59-62, 64, 66, 67, 69-73, 75, 76-79, 82-85, 101, 102, 103, 106-115

Asthma 81

Autoimmune 11-13, 20, 21, 24, 25, 35, 36, 41, 42, 102, 109, 110

Bacillus 82, 84, 85, 86

Bacteria 65, 78, 82, 85

Bile 22, 25, 26, 32, 37, 44, 52, 53-55, 66, 84, 108

Bilirubin 20, 25, 37, 39, 53, 55, 85, 106, 113, 114

Biopsy 8, 11, 21, 24, 95, 101, 112

Bleeding 20, 38, 40, 43, 44, 70, 86, 112, 113

Blood-clotting 43

Blood-lipid-reduction 63

Blood rheology 36, 57, 58

Blood stagnancy 26, 36, 58

Blood-sugar-regulating 62, 63, 84

BM Capsule 42

Bronchitis 42, 65, 81, 85

CAH (chronic active hepatitis) 19, 20

Calcium 55, 72, 78

Calories 99

Cancer 4, 17, 70, 81, 114

Candidiasis 85

Capillaris Combination 37, 66, 67

Carbon tetrachloride 47, 48, 74

Carcinoma 4

Cardiomyopathy 112

Cardiovascular 60, 82, 85

Chemotherapy 12, 76, 81, 98

Chickenpox 57

Circulation Tablet No. 1 34, 57, 58, 59, 113

Circulation Tablet No. 4 39, 59

Cholagogic 52, 53, 54, 66, 84

Cholangitis 53

Cholelithiasis 54

Choleretic 52, 53, 54, 66

Cholestatic 66

Cholesterol 53, 55, 80

CIC (circulatory immunocomplex) 25, 27

Cirrhosis 3, 4, 13, 16, 17, 19, 21, 23, 26, 27, 28, 38, 43, 50, 59, 61, 74, 75, 80, 89, 93, 94, 101, 103, 112, 114

Co-infection 8

Colitis 20, 70

Collagen 27, 50, 62, 76, 94

Conjunctiva 55, 93, 107, 110

Constipation 57, 86

Contraindicated 13, 33, 104

Coptin 42, 43, 84, 85, 90

Coptin Tablet 44, 84

Cordyceps 25, 27, 36, 38-40, 79-81, 90, 94, 113

Cordyceps Capsule 36, 79, 113

Cortico-steroids 70, 65, 74

CPH (chronic persistent hepatitis) 19, 20

Cryoglobulinemia 25, 35

Cytochrome 51

Cytonecrosis 50

Cytopathic 24, 35, 94

Cytopenias 13

Decompensation 13, 99, 111

Depression 11, 13, 71, 72, 102, 105

Detoxification 48, 52, 64, 73, 78, 98, 99

Dextran 50, 58

Diabetes 32, 35, 40, 41, 42, 62, 63, 85, 112

Diarrhea 44, 68, 102, 103, 105, 106, 110, 113

DIC (diffused intra-vascular clotting) 58

Diet 98, 99, 101, 103

Dimethoxycoumarin 53

Disorientation 112

Displasia 111

Diuretic 69

Dizziness 11, 75

DNA 90, 95, 97

DNAP (DNA polymerase) 90

Dysentery 82, 85

Eczema 65

Edema 20, 40, 43, 61, 69, 75, 107, 111

Emaciation 68

Encephalitis 56, 57

Esophagus 38, 43, 61, 112

Etiologic 12, 31

Exercise 5, 100

Fat 8, 47, 50, 53, 97

Fatigue 8, 11, 20-22, 24, 32, 40, 71, 76, 100, 102, 103, 105, 106

Fever 20, 105, 106

Fibroblastic 20, 27

Fibrolytic 54

Fibrosis 8, 16, 17, 19, 23, 25, 26, 32, 37-39, 49, 50, 57, 59, 61, 74, 94

Fungi 82

Galactosamine 52

Gall 25, 37, 52, 55, 66, 108, 113

Gallbladder 25, 26, 37, 53, 54, 55, 67, 85, 86

Gall Formula No. 1 37, 52, 113

Gallstones 8, 25, 26, 37, 54, 55

Gammaglobulin 20, 25, 50, 74

Garlic 42, 82, 83

Gastritis 68, 70, 85, 86

Genipin 53

GGT 25, 37, 39, 55, 107-113

Ginger 47, 49

Ginseng 44, 67, 68

Ginseng & Atractylodes Formula 44, 67, 68

Globulinemia 35

Glucocorticoid 74

Glucose 41, 63

Glycogen 41, 47, 48, 54, 67, 74, 76

Glycyrrhizin (GL) 24, 27, 33, 34-36, 38, 72-75, 88, 89, 91, 94, 102, 110, 115

Glycyrrhizin Capsule 33, 75, 88, 91, 102, 110, 115

GMP 46

Granuloma 59

Group I 34, 89, 93, 115

Group II 34, 89, 93

HBAg 56
HBcAg 22
HBeAb 108
HBeAg 22, 73, 107, 108
HBsAg 15, 22, 48, 90, 107
HBV 16, 22, 87, 89, 90, 91, 105, 108
HBV-DNA 22
HBV-DNAP 22
HCV 4, 12, 13, 16, 17, 18, 22, 24, 26-29, 31, 32, 34, 35, 36, 41, 42, 56, 57, 87, 89, 91, 94, 95-98, 101, 102, 105, 111, 115
HCV RNA PCR 91, 95, 101, 115
HDL 80
Hemorrhaging 57
Hemorrhoids 38, 61
Hepa Formula No. 2 23, 24, 33, 47, 89, 102, 110
Hepa Formula No. 3 39, 49, 92, 113
Hepa Formula No. 4 39, 51
HerbSom 41, 60
HerbSom Capsule 41, 60
HerbZac 71
HerbZac Capsule 71
Herpes 1, 56, 77, 78, 90
Histamine 65, 74
Histological 10, 19, 20, 47, 53, 67, 74, 95
HIV 1, 4, 7, 8, 18, 30, 77, 78, 90, 97, 105
Homeostatic 70, 86
Humeral immunity 25, 35, 59

Hypertension 33, 37, 43, 61, 75, 81, 85
Hyperthyroidism 13
Hypertrophy 20, 26, 67
Hypoglycemia 62, 63
Hypothyroidism 110, 111

Icterohepatitis 76
IFN (interferon) 2, 8, 9, 11, 12, 13-16, 28, 29, 96, 97, 98, 103-105, 109, 110, 112
IFN-resistant 96
Immune-regulatory 21, 25, 52, 76, 86
Immunopathic 24, 35, 41, 94
Indigestion 57
Influenza 56, 57, 77, 78, 84
Insomnia 11, 22, 32, 40, 41, 60
Insulin 42, 63
Interferon-gamma 73
Iron 72
ITP (idiopathic thrombocytopenia) 69, 109, 110

Jaundice 8, 16, 20, 21, 25, 26, 37, 53-56, 66, 67, 76, 97, 107, 108

Kidney 75, 76, 79, 91, 99
Kupffer cell 58

LDH 48
Leukemia 64, 78
Leukopenia 52, 56, 76
Leukorrhea 81

LFTs (liver function tests) 105,
    106, 107, 108
Libido 81
Licorice 24, 25, 47, 49, 51, 72,
    73, 75
Ligustrin 33, 75, 76, 88, 89,
    102, 110, 113, 115
Ligustrin Capsule 33, 75, 88,
    89, 102, 110, 113, 115
Linolenic acid 75
Lipids 54
Lipoproteins 80, 81
Lithogogic 54, 55
Liver Failure 17, 112, 114
Liver Palm 20, 26, 58, 112
Lymphoblast 76

Macrophages 58, 59, 76, 80
Malaise 11, 105
MCM (modern Chinese
    medicine), 7
Meditation 100
MHV 73
Microcirculation 16, 22, 26, 27,
    32, 36, 37, 49, 50, 57, 58
Mycobacteria 82,84

Necrosis 20, 51, 53, 67, 74, 75
Nephritis 20, 68, 69
Neurodermatitis 65
Newcastle virus 78, 84
Non-responders 13, 24
Nucleoside 12, 97, 98
Nutrition 19, 37, 38, 98

Oleanolic acid 23, 75
Oleaolic acid 33
Oleuopein 77, 78
Oliguria 66
Olive leaf 22, 35, 64, 77, 78, 79,
    90
Olivessence Capsule 35, 78
Osmotic pressure 43, 94
Oxymatrine 51, 56
Ozone 102, 103

Painkillers 99
Pancreas 42, 63, 86
Pancreatitis 68
Peony 38, 61, 69
Phagocytosis 58, 59, 76, 80
Platelet 43, 57, 58 70, 80, 104,
    109-112, 114
Polio 78
Polymerase 22, 90
Portal vein 20, 32, 37, 38, 43,
    61, 81, 93
Potassium 33, 34, 72, 75
Prednisone 109
Pregnant 64
Prognosis 2, 19, 23, 89
Protozoa 78, 82, 85
Psoriasis 35, 40, 41, 112-114
Psoriatic 112, 114
Psychiatric 12, 98
PTT 58, 114

Qi 16, 68, 72, 79
Qi-gong 5, 100

Rashes 20, 22, 25, 32, 35, 40, 41, 58, 73

Rebetron 12-14, 27, 98, 110

Red Peony Capsule 38

Relapse 11, 13, 109, 110

Rheumatism 65, 69

Rhubarb 43, 85, 86

Rhubarbin 42, 43, 85, 86

Rhubarbin Tablet 42, 43, 85, 86

Ribavirin 12, 15, 16, 28, 97, 98, 110

Ritalin 102, 103

RNA 18, 54, 67, 74, 91, 97, 115

Sandy stone 54, 55

Selenium 99

SGPT (see ALT)

SGOT (see AST)

Silicosis 27, 61, 62, 94

Spider mole 20, 26, 58, 93, 94, 112

Spleen 20, 26, 38, 59, 61, 73, 80, 93, 94, 111, 113, 114

Steatosis 50

Stephania & Astragalus Combination 43, 69

Stress 35, 95, 102, 103

Synthroid 109

TCM (Traditional Chinese Medicine) 4-7, 10, 11, 14, 16, 27, 28, 30, 36, 45, 46, 49, 52, 53, 56, 58, 60, 64-66, 72, 73, 77-79

Thrombocytopenia 57, 104, 109

Thyroid 20, 35, 109-111

Tinnitus 75

Tonsillitis 85

Toxicity 7, 39, 65, 76, 80, 85, 86, 91

Transplant 13, 17, 21, 55, 94, 105, 112, 115

Tuberculosis 81, 82, 84

Ulcerative colitis 20, 68, 70, 73

Ulcers 65, 92

Varices 38, 43, 61, 93, 111

Vasculitis 20, 25, 35, 40, 41

Virostatic 22, 35, 56, 57, 66

Virus 3, 13, 18, 19, 22, 24, 25, 27, 29, 30, 56, 57, 73, 84, 87, 89, 90, 91, 94, 96, 107, 109

WBC 76

Yeast 85

Yunnan paiyao 44, 70, 113